Democratic Governance and Health

Democratic Governance and Health: Hospitals, Politics and Health Policy in New Zealand

MIRIAM J. **LAUGESEN** & ROBIN **GAULD**

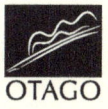

OTAGO

Miriam J. Laugesen would like to dedicate this book
to her parents, Helen Glasgow and Murray Laugesen.

Robin Gauld would like to dedicate this book to his parents,
John and Alison Gauld and, of course, to his wife, Ina Bercinskas
and children, Edward and Honor.

Published by Otago University Press
Level 1 / 398 Cumberland Street
PO Box 56, Dunedin, New Zealand
Email: university.press@otago.ac.nz
Fax: 64 3 479 8385
www.otago.ac.nz/press

First published 2012

ISBN 978 1 877578 27 4

Publisher: Wendy Harrex
Editing and type design: Georgina McWhirter
Cover design: Fiona Moffat
Index: Diane Lowther

Cover: 'Demonstrators with banners, during a march protesting against the closure of Elderslea Maternity Hospital in Upper Hutt'. Photograph taken by Ray Pigney, *Dominion Post*. Ref: EP/1989/4141/12. Alexander Turnbull Library, Wellington, New Zealand.

Printed in Wellington, New Zealand, by Printstop Ltd

Contents

Acronyms

AHB: Area Health Board
BMA: British Medical Association
CCMAU: Crown Company
Monitoring Advisory Unit
CHE: Crown Health Enterprise
DHB: District Health Board
GP: General Practitioner
HBA: Hospital Boards' Association
HFA: Health Funding Authority
HHS: Hospital and Health Service
MANZ: Medical Association of New Zealand
MMP: Mixed Member Proportional
MP: Member of Parliament
NHB: National Health Board
NHS: National Health Service
PBF: Population-Based Funding
PHO: Primary Health Organisation
RHA: Regional Health Authority
SACHSO: Special Advisory Committee
on Health Services Organisation
SOE: State-Owned Enterprise
STV: Single Transferrable Vote
THA: Transitional Health Authority

Acknowledgements

THIS BOOK arose from a chance discussion between the authors over lunch at a Dominican restaurant near the Columbia University Medical Center campus in mid-2010. Shortly after Robin returned to New Zealand, we decided to tackle this project together. Combining forces, we produced a book different but arguably stronger than we could have written separately, and the process was one of pleasant and collaborative authorial partnership.

We are grateful for the funding that made the research and production of this book possible, the Health Research Council of New Zealand's grant to Miriam Laugesen (Post-Graduate Grant 96-405); the University of Melbourne; and Columbia University's Department of Health Policy and Management for staff support for editorial work on the book. Many organisations and individuals facilitated the research, including Evelina Pereira and records staff of the Ministry of Health; National Archives staff; David Reitter and staff at the Alexander Turnbull Library, and the New Zealand Medical Association. UMR Insight, Television New Zealand, Jack Vowles, Nigel Roberts, and the Australian National University Data Archive provided public opinion data and assistance.

Samantha Gilman provided conscientious and patient compilation of the references and copy-edited the manuscript. We are grateful also to Wendy Harrex, Georgina McWhirter, Diane Lowther and the staff at Otago University Press for their work in bringing the book to publication. Peter Davis gave us excellent suggestions on the manuscript and Geoff Fougere gave us detailed and insightful comments on the final draft. It is greatly improved as a result. Finally, intellectually, we benefited (at different times) from the wisdom imparted by Robert Gregory and John Martin when we were students at Victoria University of Wellington.

Miriam Laugesen thanks Elizabeth McLeay for inspiration and intellectual dedication to the project from the beginning. Brian Galligan and Bruce Headey were key mentors; and Carolyn Hughes Tuohy and Jack Nagel read earlier versions of chapters. For everything from practical editorial help, to providing a place to stay, or for loyal friendship, she is grateful to Antong Victorio, Alisa Hirschfeld, Ben Berger, Alan Jacobs, Jim and Mary Barr, Ashley Cox, Alex Frankel, Paola Bilbrough, Eddie Miller, Kate Robb, Karen Farquharson, Tim Marjoribanks, Helen and Neville Glasgow, Murray Laugesen, Mark Laugesen, Ruth Laugesen and Red Yska, and Jocelyn Keith. Last but not least, Andy Sabl supported this project in so many ways, from its early beginnings through to the end.

Robin Gauld thanks colleagues in the Department of Preventive and Social Medicine, University of Otago, for encouraging and supporting his efforts over the years to research the New Zealand health system and especially the DHBs, and the University of Otago for various research grants.

Miriam J. Laugesen
June, 2012, New York, USA

Robin Gauld
June, 2012, Dunedin, New Zealand

CHAPTER **ONE**

Democratic governance and health: an introduction

'Our hospital board system has been described as being politically controlled ... It is public control by elective boards under departmental supervision and assistance. It is a true expression of our democratic free institutions.' – Minister of Health, 1926

NEW ZEALAND is the only country in the world where elected health boards have been a core and enduring feature of the governance arrangements for health care in the post-war period. Elected boards have survived the ongoing health system reform attempts that have occurred from across the political spectrum, usually in the wake of elections and changes of government. Though some changes to governance and planning structures in the late 1980s succeeded, elected boards have remained largely untouched since the nineteenth century. One exception was the 1990s, when the government removed elected boards and attempted to establish a market-oriented health service. Based on previous failures, political leaders thought elected boards could only be removed if it was done without any prior warning, and swiftly. Ironically, the effect of introducing a dramatic agenda of reform in the 1990s was that government over-reached, leading voters and health care professionals to reject the health reform programme, which created the momentum for subsequent policy reversals. From 2000–01, a new government reintroduced elected representation in the health care system through the creation of District Health Boards (DHBs), confirming the stubborn resilience of the hospital board model.

Governments and health systems around the world are increasingly promoting public participation in health care decision-making (Wait and Nolte, 2006), for a variety of reasons. Participation can build support for increasingly complex decisions about resource allocation, service location and service configuration; embed decision-making structures in local communities and promote community partnership and engagement; enable decision-makers to learn more from the public and specific communities about their preferences and needs; and bring an element of transparency and public accountability to health care planning and decision-making. Elected boards could increase health system legitimacy. Such boards are only one of a variety of methods for involving the public in decision-making, yet they remain both conceptually important and aspirational for policy-makers and communities in many parts of the world who are grappling with how to increase public participation in health care.

A few Canadian provinces briefly experimented with elected boards, but New Zealand's experience is unique. As a result, research on how elected boards are constructed, and how they function and perform is unusual. Being a small country, there are fewer researchers with a sustained interest in elected health boards and their performance; New Zealanders have tended to take this aspect of the health care system for granted. This is surprising, given the influence of elected boards historically. In 2011, the (predominantly) elected boards were responsible for much of the $12 billion in public expenditure directly funded by the taxpayers via the Ministry of Health. These boards also made all major decisions regarding how health services are configured in the areas they serve, including which services are to be funded, for whom and where they should be located.

Democratic Governance and Health seeks to fill a gap in the literature by providing a comprehensive examination of the development of New Zealand's elected health boards from the 1930s to the present DHB structure. We analyse the history of democratic governance of health care, how New Zealand's boards have functioned, the politics surrounding reform of elected boards, and explore the idea of local democracy and health care decision-making. Based on extensive primary research of historical and other sources, we take a critical look at the capacity of elected boards to effectively govern the allocation and management of public expenditure on behalf of the taxpayer and patients. This approach is called the 'realist' view of public participation. Elected boards and the realities of public participation fall short of expectations in several ways. The chapters that follow show the elected governance structures have:

- Created an institutional arrangement that local communities have rallied around when threatened, making it politically difficult for central government to reconfigure them.
- Been vessels for promoting national party-political goals as well as local political goals, and not necessarily those that will best benefit the public and patients.
- Assumed a symbolic role in communities taking a last-stand against marketisation of New Zealand health care and been both embraced and defended by national political elites who signal their opposition to market models.
- Possibly failed to provide the skill set demanded for effective health-care planning, decision-making and financial management.
- Failed to garner public attention at election time, while simultaneously rally-crying when threatened, bringing into question their legitimacy.

Through an historical journey of local health system governance we find there is a strong element of path dependence in the institutional arrangements and policies of the New Zealand health system. Path dependence is the theory that policy change is influenced by pre-existing policy arrangements that are deeply embedded (Pierson, 2002; Wilsford, 1994). The ways people within the system work with one another, the expectations they have about the system and how services are governed, funded, and organised, become entrenched over time, especially in a large and complex system such as national health care. Organisations become institutionalised and, over time, become institutions. Institutions have historical roots because they are the residue of past actions and choices that embody, preserve and impart differential power resources with respect to different individuals and groups (Klein, 1996). Political conflicts are fought out by groups that were formed within distinctive political structures with a long history (Immergut, 1992). Path dependency means that policy changes are made where change is likely to be politically achievable (goals will be acceptable to the range of institutions and interests) and technically achievable (changes will not completely disrupt service continuity). These may include small changes at the margins of the system, such as attempts to better organise planning amongst DHB regions, or the creation of new national arrangements to promote improvements in quality and patient safety. 'Incrementalism' is an appropriate description for this kind of policy change and it refers to 'what is possible' in policy-making and change.

Given the restrictions of path dependency and interest groups, it provides an explanation of how core policies and organisational arrangements are sustained over time with only minimal change occurring (Lindblom, 1959). Incrementalism, by its very name, suggests that policy changes tend to be minor and built upon existing arrangements. Both path dependency and incrementalism have influenced the development of New Zealand's system of health service governance and the present DHB structure.

As in most developed countries, where hospitals usually consume the largest share of health expenditure, hospitals in New Zealand have been the main focus for reducing the cost of health care. Health expenditure has been growing at a rate often considered by political leaders and analysts to be unsustainable. Among Organization for the Economic Cooperation and Development (OECD) member countries, it has been increasing at twice the general rate of inflation since at least the mid-1990s (OECD, 2009). In New Zealand, health expenditure increased from 8 per cent of Gross Domestic Product (GDP) in 2000 to 9.2 per cent in 2011. The public sector is increasingly responsible for the health care needs of New Zealanders: public expenditure on health doubled throughout the decade of the 2000s in real terms. Today the government funds just over 80 per cent of total health expenditure. Other than the United States, governments of higher-income OECD countries typically finance around 70 per cent of total health expenditure (OECD, 2009). While no country has developed a formula for reducing or containing the expenditure increases, all are focused on efficiency and improved performance.

'Performance' is a challenging concept because it can be analysed in different ways, it has different meanings to different groups (Smith et al., 2009) and there are many distinct components. We can measure financial performance through the study of routine budget data but working out how well a DHB or other government-funded provider is performing in other areas can be complex. DHBs are financed using a population-based funding formula, which means some are in a perpetual state of 'deficit' (some would say 'underfunded'). A sub-optimal financial performance may simply be due to inadequate funding. Other elements of performance may include 'responsiveness' to communities, accountability both to local electors and to central government demands, achievement of policy objectives, and the basic capacity to govern and steer both the local DHB and public hospital and health care services. On the last point, this book considers whether DHB boards are in front of driving quality improvement, including system design for error reduction, reducing clinical practice variation and improving patient flow.

The conclusion discusses whether the electoral model is superior to the model used in countries where boards are, almost without exception, composed of appointees. Lessons are drawn from the periods when boards were dominant, as well as periods when they were not. The demise of the elected board structure in New Zealand in the 1990s provides a rich source of information to draw upon. Both Chapter Five and our previous work (Gauld, 2000; Gauld, 2001; Laugesen, 2005) show why the competitive market model of the early 1990s failed. There is no evidence that appointed boards and generic managers performed any better than elected boards. The latter part of the 1990s featured appointed boards and a corporate governance model, but within a national framework designed to address flaws in the competitive market model. By the end of the decade, boards showed improved performance, but national policy changes could have been the cause. If the appointed or managerial models fail to represent unequivocal alternatives, how might the electoral model be improved upon? The concluding chapter provides some suggestions.

The historical resilience of New Zealand's health boards

The New Zealand health care system has remained stubbornly resistant to government attempts to remove elections from local hospital or health boards for over a century. In every reform episode (Table 1) from the 1920s through to the present DHB system, governments tried but failed to overturn elected boards. Subsequent chapters explain how central government was constrained by elected hospital boards that were simultaneously providers of health care and institutions of representation (except during the 1990s). Governments had two relatively consistent objectives: to change hospital board representation and to regionalise small, local hospitals. Successive governments hoped changes to both would give them more control over the health sector. However, they have struggled in vain to reform the sector. Regionalisation was finally forced on hospital boards in 1989 when the Labour Government established a system of fourteen Area Health Boards that replaced thirty-seven hospital boards. Changes to representation proved the hardest to manoeuvre and attempts failed until 1991. Cabinet used the passage of the budget and parliamentary rules of urgency to (literally) disband elected boards overnight. Then,

Table 1. Episodes of hospital reform and outcomes

Reform episode	Policy recommendation	Outcome
1928s–32	A Board of Hospitals to manage the hospital system.	No change
Social Security Act 1935–42	Health benefits for primary and hospital care; few changes to hospitals.	*Laissez-faire* hospital financing policies.
Commission on Hospital Reform 1952–53	Some appointment of board members; five regional health authorities, more accountability.	1957 legislation did not change hospital governance.
Royal Commission on Hospital Services 1971–72	Commission abolished	Commission was abolished because of change in government.
Labour Caucus Committee 1972–75	Change elected representation; regional base hospitals.	No policy change
Special Advisory Committee on Hospital System Organisation 1976–84	Change elected representation; regional health boards.	Voluntary regionalisation policy
Health Benefits Review, 1986–87	Regional Area Health Boards	See below
Hospital and Related Services Taskforce 1987–90	Six regional health authorities; elected members; role for competition in provision/ internal market.	Indirectly led to the 1989 Area Health Boards Act, which compels hospital boards to restructure into 14 boards from 29.
Health Services Taskforce 1991–93	Abolish Area Health Boards and elected representation; regional purchasing; competition in provision and financing.	Representation abolished, quasi-internal market established until 1996, four regional purchasers, one national purchaser 1996.
1996–2000	Coalition agreement of 1996 starts process towards single national Health Funding Authority.	Reduce commercial emphasis in health care and move back in the direction of local control of health care.
2000–10	Create DHBs with elected epresentation and local planning and purchasing responsibilities.	DHBs in place but questions about performance and adequacy of model.

elected District Health Boards were reinstated in 2000.

Time and again reformers believed they would succeed in reorganising health boards but success has tended to be elusive, partly because of the path-dependent nature of these structures: 'local autonomy has proved to be a stronger influence in health services organisation', writes Brunton (1983, p.4). Hospital boards had deep roots – shaped by colonial patterns of population distribution – which were dispersed. Many hospitals were established during the gold rush of the late nineteenth century, in remote areas.

Hospital boards were first formally constituted by the 1885 Hospital and Charitable Institutions Act. Hospital boards established under the legislation were body corporates, and were capable of holding real and personal property. The Act was based on three principles: that committees of hospital management should be essentially local and made amenable to public opinion by being elected, expenditure should be localised, and central government should meet a reasonable proportion of expenditure but it should not be the funder of the last resort (Department of Health, 1975). Hospital districts (which formed the geographical and electoral basis for hospital boards) were comprised of one or more counties and boroughs, and town districts within the boundaries of a county or counties. In the early 1950s, districts varied from 2800 people to Auckland's 378,000 residents (Statistics New Zealand, 1951), with urban areas rapidly growing in size while rural districts suffered declines or plateaux in population. Unlike electoral districts, hospital districts were not subject to re-districting according to population. District population disparities were irritating to central government bureaucrats and ministers, and the inverse relationship between population and hospital districts itself is a demonstration of the historical roots of hospital boards and their autonomy.

Revisions of the 1885 Hospitals and Charitable Institutions legislation took place in 1909, 1926, and 1957, when the Hospitals Act replaced the 1885 legislation. Despite revisions and eventual replacement, the 1885 legislation set the tone of central–local relationships that only slowly allowed greater ministerial control. The 1885 Act specified that hospitals would have exclusive 'superintendence' and 'control' of their institutions. In 1909, this was modified slightly to specify 'control and management'. The 1885 legislation allowed boards to establish hospitals in their district. This remained constant through the first half of the twentieth century. In the early 1950s, hospital boards were responsible for establishing, controlling and managing a range of institutions, including hospitals, maternity and convalescent homes, institutions for alcoholics and sanatoria (Statistics New Zealand, 1951). However, boards could not borrow money for building establishment or land purchases, capital expenditure or debt servicing in the 1950s. Boards were required to submit estimates of expenditure for capital and maintenance purposes and to confirm the estimates at a special board meeting. The minister could require boards to amend the estimate submitted (Statistics New Zealand, 1951). Boards were also limited in their expenditure on land, building or other capital items to purchases less than £250, and could not sell or exchange land or close an institution. By 1957, hospital boards required the minister's prior consent to open hospitals.

Hospital boards were not constrained by statutes relating to the medical services they should provide, except in relation to infectious diseases. From the earliest days, discretion mainly lay with hospitals to provide medical and other care. In 1885, hospitals were required to admit any sufferer of infectious disease if the Chief Health Officer directed admission. By amendment in 1909, and in 1957, the legislation specified that admission to hospitals was only required if accommodation was available. This requirement meant that boards would have had few incentives to provide more with fewer resources. By 1970, hospital boards were required to provide medical services and facilities that were specified by the Minister of Health, but the norm of service being conditional on existing resources had arguably become customary.

In the second half of the twentieth century, changing population distribution brought differences in hospital boards' size and resources into sharp relief. The population shifted towards the North Island, but there were more boards located in the South Island than the North. In 1961, around 60 per cent of hospital boards were located in the South Island, even though only 30 per cent of the population lived there. In 1986, only 26 per cent of the population lived in the South Island, while the South retained 41 per cent of the nation's hospital boards. Population increases in the North Island were concentrated in the Auckland metropolitan area. By 1994, almost 38 per cent of New Zealanders lived in the Auckland regional council area. These figures are only an indication of the concentration of population in the metro Auckland area rather than across time comparisons. Area boundaries for 1991 and 1983 are slightly different so should not be used for comparison. As a result, boards contained very different numbers of people. In the early 1950s, districts varied from 2800 people to 378,000

Table 2. New Zealand hospital/health board numbers, 1925–2011

Year	No. of Boards
1925	46
1935	45
1940	42
1951	37
1960	37
1970	31
1975	29
1980	29
1985	29
1988	29
1989	14
1991	23*
2000	21
2010	20

Note: all boards feature elected members except *
Source: Data from 1925–60 from Bloomfield (1984). Data from 1961–88 compiled from various Department of Health volumes (1961–88).

(Auckland) (Statistics New Zealand, 1951), with urban areas rapidly growing in size while rural districts suffered declines or plateaux in population. Unlike electoral districts, hospital districts were not subject to re-districting according to population.

Prior to 1957, boards could have as many as twenty members. After the 1957 Hospitals Act was passed, the maximum number of members was fourteen, with a minimum of eight. While the Hospitals Act covered many of the responsibilities of hospitals and relations between hospital boards and ministers, the legislation relating to elections was controlled by local government regulations. Hospital board members were elected in local government elections that were held every three years on a fixed date. Voting in hospital board elections was limited to property owners during some periods of the twentieth century, and at other times opened to registered voters. Turnout in local elections was never particularly high. On average, half of registered voters voted between 1970 and 1986 (Bush, 1992).

Hospital board members had weak ties to political parties. Most candidates stood for office as independents (Bush, 1992). Hospital board meetings were public and open to the press. Manifestos and political positions were largely absent in hospital board elections (Mulgan, 1984, p.123). This lessened accountability in local government, as voters found it difficult to link policies to individual members (rather than parties) (Mulgan, 1984). The professions, such as lawyers, doctors and accountants, were over-represented on hospital boards. Hospital board members had weak ties to organised groups such as the professional associations or unions, although doctors often served on hospital boards. An important incentive for serving on hospital boards was that it was an entrée into local politics and board members got visibility from which to launch their future political aspirations.

Hospital boards organised themselves nationally through the Hospital Boards' Association. The Association did not, however, act as the main and only intermediary between boards and governments during reform periods. Boards were united through their Association but were also distinctly parochial, and politicians generally consulted individual boards when pressing for reform. The lack of unity or single organisation representing hospital boards nationally may have been a result of very different interests between boards, such as the small provincial hospital boards and large metropolitan boards. On the other hand, individual negotiation may have reflected the electoral incentives politicians faced within each hospital board area. The issue of hospital board political power is discussed below.

The political power of hospital boards

The portrait above shows boards were long-established political actors within the New Zealand health system. They became institutionalised by virtue of a combination of factors. First, their influence on health policy arose from the timing of the establishment of hospital boards and their geographic distribution throughout New Zealand, influenced by colonial settlement patterns. The timing of the establishment of hospital boards allowed them to make significant gains in the absence of other alternatives. Hospital boards evolved during a period in the late nineteenth century when local, provincial and national governmental roles were being defined, and before the advent of the twentieth-century welfare state.

Second, boards became integrated into New Zealand's national health service after 1938, but funding to make hospitals free to the public was added to an existing framework of local governance and control. Hospital boards were already established as relatively independent (despite receiving government funds prior to 1938) and autonomously governed by elected representatives. The Labour Government had to work within the framework of existing institutions in 1938, when it established hospital benefits. Labour saw opening access to public hospitals as being a simple matter of increasing funding to hospitals, but the government did not give itself more say over the hospital system and Labour's Social Security Act did not change hospital governance. Nor did Labour impose constraints on hospitals as such. Boards received more money but did not have to make changes to their organisations (Condliffe, 1959). Although ministerial control over hospital boards did increase, boards retained autonomy and national funding. Hospitals did have to make some concessions in 1957 in exchange for more oversight by the Minister of Health under the Hospitals Act, but still retained a large degree of control and maintained elected representation. This created difficulties, since the health system was nationalised but not coordinated. A similar problem continues in the present DHB system, which undermines a focus on developing a high-performance health care system.

These two factors, the timing of establishment and New Zealand's settlement patterns, combined with a lack of control imposed in exchange for increased funding in 1938, contributed to make hospital boards relatively autonomous. However, these factors do not fully account for the endurance of local boards. It is possible for policies and institutions to be overcome, as the boards eventually were, in 1991. The other important aspects of hospital boards' power were more symbolic and pragmatic, and are discussed next.

Hospital boards represented an ethos of democratic representation and were closely associated with local hospitals within each community. Ideas and core political values played a role in the longevity of the hospital boards and their seeming monopoly in hospital policy. The normative ideal of democratic representation and hospital boards' close identification to the business of providing local health care gave hospital boards the legitimacy that made reform difficult. Hospital boards endured because they embodied community values of democracy and care of the sick. The role of hospital boards in fulfilling representational functions and caring for the sick helped hospital boards gain legitimacy in voters' minds.

The symbolic aspects of local boards had consequences for politics surrounding hospital reform and the incentives political actors faced.

When politicians or bureaucrats wanted more efficiency through regionalisation, or more political control through more appointed board members, these symbolic factors influenced their political options and strategies. Throughout the period covered in this book, politicians in central government found that board reform was potentially costly politically. A policy that imposes losses on specific constituencies, while distributing benefits widely, is inherently difficult for politicians (Pierson, 1994). Some types of hospital reform were potentially more costly than other policies. Hospital closure was the most risky of all possible policies; so was hospital regionalisation and changes to hospital boards composition. The visibility of policy measures and their traceability to the average voter has been shown to be important in analysing congressional voting in the United States (Arnold, 1990). A similar dynamic operates in all legislative settings. In all legislatures, the magnitude of the costs and benefits in a policy change, the timing, the proximity to voters and the availability of an instigator to reveal citizens' stakes in the outcome, all determine the electoral influence of any government policy (Arnold, 1990). In every electorate, hospital boards could rally against health care reform.

Governance: what is it and why is it important?

Over the past decade or so, 'governance' has been of increasing importance in the health care policy agenda both in New Zealand and internationally, although there is nothing conceptually new about it (Rhodes, 1997). Here, governance refers to the arrangements for governing the organisation and management of health services. Governance is associated with various other concepts such as oversight, steering and providing strategic direction through policy development or approval, ensuring that services are well managed and by the right people, and scrutiny through demanding that service providers are accountable for various aspects of performance. As such, governance has the potential to make a difference between a high-performing health system and one that is mediocre.

Health systems are complex, and usually comprised of a variety of organisational forms (large public and private bureaucracies, small businesses, networks and non-government organisations). Effective governance is challenging. Focusing primarily on the bottom line, as directors of private companies might, is unlikely to produce strong results. The health care governance role, particularly in a public system such as New Zealand, requires in-depth understanding of an array of services and issues:

public financial management and accounting, clinical services ranging from primary care to surgery, how the various pieces of the system fit together, technology and support services, national and international trends, and innovations in health care delivery. A governing body also needs to be able to gain the confidence of health care providers and so the board requires strong communication skills.

Models of governance: corporate, market, democratic and clinical

A committee or board generally leads with the support of a full-time secretariat. This will most likely include a chief executive officer and other support staff who oversee an organisation such as a hospital or other health services. This can lead to tensions (Goold and Campbell, 1987; Perrow, 1986). A board and management can disagree on organisational directions. Full-time officials may have considerably more information on issues than the board, leading to situations where the board is manipulated, is unable to provide adequate scrutiny, and simply 'rubber stamps' managerial decisions. Public sector boards, such as DHBs, may be under considerable external 'shareholder' pressure (ministers being the shareholders as such), in turn placing demands on officials to perform in particular ways that may appear counter-intuitive.

Depending on the philosophical predisposition of political leaders, governing boards in the public sector may be constituted differently. Under the influence of a more managerialist model, in which private business skills are seen as critical to effective public management, a 'corporate' structure would be comprised of appointed members drawn mainly from the private business sector. Board meetings are usually held in private, with limited consultation of public and professional groups, and there is a greater emphasis on financial performance and service efficiency. Formal contracts and financial incentives are often used to improve staff performance. This was the model adopted in New Zealand in the 1990s.

At the opposite end of the spectrum, a democratic or community-oriented board structure may feature elected members with a goal of bringing community input into the decision-making process. If there are appointees, they may be selected for their experience in community work, connectedness to community or other groups such as representatives of the medical or other professions, or for specific skills in governance. Meetings may be open to the public to promote transparency, and there is likely to be considerable consultation to ensure that the perspectives of different groups and service providers are incorporated. In the contemporary environment, contracts and incentives are still likely to be central to driving performance. This is simply a function of the overlap of both managerial and democratic perspectives on governance and organisational performance (Gauld, 2009).

Compared with the private sector, governance in the public sector is particularly complex (Lane, 1995). Central government may provide the overarching strategic policy directions, while local or professionally based governing bodies work through the detail of developing specific policy responses, creating accountability structures and performance monitoring. Governance is not a strictly 'top-down' arrangement that is controlled and administered by central government: instead this is a model of devolution. This type of structure, used in the New Zealand DHB system, is characterised by a complicated web of decision-making structures. This requires substantial negotiation and communication both vertically, between central government and the local governance level, as well as horizontally, amongst the various local boards. Under this model, elements of the corporate management model and competitive markets are layered onto a model of devolution. Local boards may be required to both compete with one another around certain tasks, such as targets for service delivery, while also collaborating to ensure consistent implementation of national policy directions such as equity of service access.

Both corporate or democratic governance models may include health professional representation. This is similar to a traditional hospital management model where doctors or nurses managed hospitals. This traditional approach weakened through the 1980s and 1990s, when the more purist version of the corporate governance model was adopted. However, a resurgence of interest in the concept and practice of 'clinical governance' (Scally and Donaldson, 1998) has occurred over the last decade, which goes beyond representation of health professionals. This model of clinical governance is different from the traditional model because today there is more awareness of the need for quality improvement and patient safety. Studies from the United States, England, Australia and New Zealand indicate that up to 12 per cent of hospital patients will be the victim of an error in the process of their care (Davis et al., 2002; Thomas et al., 2000; Vincent et al., 2001; Wilson et al., 1995). Common errors occur in the administration and prescribing of medicines (overdoses or wrong medicines given), while the failure to ensure adequate follow-up in post-operative care can result in a patient suffering some form of infection or complication (Leape et al., 1993). Some patients will suffer long-term disability, and others will die as a result of errors.

The incidence of medical misadventure is partly driving the focus on clinical governance in some countries. High-profile cases, such as the Shipman and Bristol Hospital Infirmary inquiries in England, have led to calls that the medical profession, in particular, has failed to adequately self-regulate. Systems have failed to ensure that professionals are competent to practice (Bristol Royal Infirmary Inquiry, 2001; Cartwright, 1988; Shipman Inquiry, 2004). This has led to a demand for more systematic and robust peer review amongst professionals, for greater public involvement and for professionals themselves to lead new professional governance processes – to drive change from within, rather than have this imposed by external forces, such as government (Irvine, 1999; Irvine, 2005).

As researchers looked for answers to the causes of low quality and medical errors they found the 'system' in which clinicians work and the processes of care explain most cases (Department of Health, 2000; Institute of Medicine, 2000; Quality Improvement Committee, 2009). For example, there may be poor communication between the clinical staff taking care of patients, and/or a lack of standard clinical processes followed by staff.

Clinical governance requires clinicians to step forward to lead the organisation and improve the delivery process and this leverages the shared training, experience and norms of clinicians. The underlying relationships of trust mean staff are more likely to learn from each other and work together to improve the organisation and delivery of clinical services, as well as being ideally placed to lead in quality and process improvement efforts.

Leadership is based on a 'small l' model; clinicians seek to lead and encourage teamwork amongst others in their specific clinical area, as opposed to the traditional approach of clinicians working as individual, autonomous professionals albeit within the context of a larger organisation (Bohmer, 2010a). Clinicians and managers are expected to collaborate through joint decision-making structures, with shared responsibility and accountability for planning and resource allocation. Clinical teams and groups work in partnership to improve the systems and processes of care, with the patients' needs and safety at the centre. The aim is to dissolve any divisions between these two groups and reduce the management–clinical hierarchies, which can create animosity and lead to organisational dysfunction. There is often a focus on the patient experience and service efficiency based on reducing gaps in the processes of care. The model features integration of primary and secondary care, as well as different services (e.g. emergency department, radiology, laboratory services).

Clinical governance activities may also be focused on reducing medical practice variation so that all patients receive exactly the same standard and procedures of care. Variation where there is no clinical justification for providing a different treatment regime for a patient remains a serious concern with considerable costs for health systems (Mulley, 2009; Wennberg, 2002), but most hospitals and health systems around the world have minimal knowledge of how much variation occurs within their own organisations. In contrast, other industries such as aviation have used the best available evidence to reduce variation in procedures to ensure safe and reliable service delivery (Lewis et al., 2011). Estimates suggest around 75 per cent of health care delivered in hospitals is routine and germane to standardised processes (Bohmer, 2010b). In the clinical governance model, clinicians work together to agree on standardised processes, which are documented and adhered to.

Should the public be involved in decision-making?

Public involvement is the aim of the democratic model that has historically dominated health governance in New Zealand, and there are many reasons for public participation. One reason for involving the public is that financing of health care is mostly from public sources, and if people are paying for health services, such as through general taxation, they should have a say in how these are shaped, as opposed to simply handing control over to corporate appointees or managers. Another argument is that diverse community preferences need a mechanism for representation, especially in situations of restricted resources where trade-offs between the funding or location of different services need to be made and community values need to be accounted for (Ham and Robert, 2003). Without representation, public views about what is best for them may not be understood by managers and health professionals making decisions behind closed doors (Florin and Dixon, 2004). Likewise, there is the argument that services improve with greater public involvement. Democratic decision-making improves public accountability and is an inherent public good (Fudge et al., 2008), since it has a potential to improve health outcomes. For example, public demand for quality improvement would improve efficiency and reduce error rates. Lastly, with public involvement in decision-making there is also the potential for increased public 'ownership' or acceptance of policies and strategic directions.

There are varying degrees to which the public might participate. Arnstein's 'ladder of participation' is potentially helpful (Arnstein, 1969). At one end of the spectrum is complete or genuine participation in which there is a full transfer of power to, and partnership with, the public. At the other end, participation may be, at best, tokenistic and likely to involve a governing body simply relaying decision-making results to the public. This model illustrates a major disadvantage of public participation: a local elected body may be used as a mechanism for central government policy-makers to deflect responsibility for making difficult decisions such as service downsizing or reconfiguration. Members of the board are placed in the unenviable position of having to explain these decisions to local constituents. Elsewhere, central government can continue to claim victory for local success stories. Other downsides of public involvement include the possibility of higher costs of the processes compared to those of appointed boards. Decision-making may be protracted in the search for commonalities and agreement amongst different groups. Balancing the various and sometimes conflicting views produced amongst different groups can be challenging for a governing body, leading to allegations that larger or more organised groups often have greater influence than do minority representatives.

The jury remains out on how best to involve the public in local decision-making (Crawford et al., 2002; Hogg, 2007). A combination of approaches may be most appropriate, including some elected representation with a mix of locally and centrally appointed members, as well as public forums, networks and meetings. Planners and decision-makers could be required to engage with the public, for example by disseminating consultation documents and inviting feedback. There is a lack of clarity about which issues need consultation and which can be made by a board. Likewise, there is no research on whether involving the public in decision-making even makes a difference to service performance and outcomes (Fudge et al., 2008; Litva et al., 2009; Litva et al., 2002). Many members of the public have limited interest in being involved in health governance issues, which is demonstrated in New Zealand and in some provinces in Canada, the two countries that have featured elections for local board members (Gauld, 2010). To offset this, it has been suggested that 'major local campaigns' may be needed to show communities how to get involved in democratic and participatory processes around health care governance (Local Government

Association Health Commission, 2008).

Despite the arguments above in favour of public involvement, there is typically a lack of clarity amongst policy-makers around the actual purposes of public involvement. If it is to improve the accountability of government, there are three types of accountability that policy-makers need to bear in mind when designing governance structures (Thorlby et al., 2008). Each has implications for the scope of public involvement, the ceding of power by a governing body and how issues will be processed. First, there is the 'giving' of an account to the public by a governing body, which may only involve reporting on activities and decisions taken. Second, is 'taking into' account public views in governance processes, which obviously provides scope for consultation, some two-way communication and even joint decision-making. Third, 'holding to' account where the local community have the power to sanction, demand answers from a governing body, and influence its activities.

An overview of the argument

To provide a broader context, Chapter Two surveys the historical development of hospital governance and health care systems in order to contrast New Zealand's development and institutional arrangements with those of other countries.

To understand participation and elected boards, we first need to understand their origins and how elected representation emerged – and persisted. Hospital reform had been an issue for New Zealand in the late nineteenth and early twentieth century and was financed from wages, local taxes, government subsidies and patient fees. Reform became even more important after the government assumed financial responsibility for hospitals. Labour's reforms, discussed in Chapter Three, gave the public free care in hospitals after 1 July 1939 and expanded the financing system beyond property owners. Hospital expenditure increased in the 1940s and hospital boards then had fewer incentives to be concerned about their expenditure. Once hospital boards realised government was paying the bill, their plans became more grandiose (Ashwin, 1956) and expenditure increased substantially. The 1953 Consultative Committee on Health Reform recommended regional health authorities to oversee hospital boards, a reduction in board numbers, and appointed rather than elected boards. Hospital boards and communities, mayors and even business associations stalled these plans. The 1957 Hospitals Act introduced few constraints on hospital boards and the 1957 Hospitals Act gave the Hospitals Advisory Council, an organisation created for hospitals (Heggie, 1969), veto power over hospital closures.

This system of local control was seriously questioned from the 1970s, discussed in Chapter Four. In 1972, the National Government established a short-lived royal commission. Labour then initiated its own reform process between 1973 and 1975. The Department of Health argued that local representation had 'perpetuated parochialism' (Department of Health, 1973). Labour's proposal was released in 1974 and also proposed a regional structure. Hospital boards were the vanguard of opposition to health care reform. Labour lost the election in 1975 and health reform became associated with electoral loss (Martin, 1991). From 1975 through to 1988 the number of hospital boards stayed constant at twenty-nine. National proceeded cautiously so it would not offend the public or hospital boards. In 1982, the government proposed to establish Area Health Boards based on population by elected and appointed officials. These proposals raised anxiety amongst hospital boards that small boards would be swallowed up by larger neighbours (National Archives). Ministers introduced a policy of voluntary regionalism in the 1983 Area Health Board Act, where boards were invited, rather than compelled, to change their organisational status. However, National's plans to reorganise hospitals along regional lines failed as few boards took up the invitation.

The new Labour Government, elected in 1984, returned to the issue of health care reform and Chapter Five discusses the growing impatience for change and the conflict between those who wanted greater hospital efficiency and those who wanted to preserve local control. Labour's experience of economic reform and state enterprises became a template for hospital reform. The 1986 Health Benefits Review was created to explore options for reorganising health benefits and begin a dialogue on system reform focused on primary care. However, Labour did not reach agreement with medical professionals over a contract scheme for primary care. In 1987, the Minister of Health appointed the Hospitals and Related Services Task Force. This Task Force quickly realised that elected hospital board members would fight any challenges to their survival. It recommended six regional health authorities that would purchase health services from the public and private sectors. The plans for reform mobilised a wide range of opponents who disagreed with commercialisation. Labour won political points for rejecting the plans and proposing a more moderate version. Labour pressed ahead with regionalism based on Area Health Boards minus the competitive market proposed by the taskforce. The new proposals seemed moderate to hospital boards when compared to the taskforce proposal. Regionalisation was finally achieved under the threat of more severe proposals for commercialisation in 1989. This arrangement was short lived, since National (elected in 1990) had its own reform plans.

The National Government built on the reviews of the 1980s when it established a new agenda for the health system in 1991 and Cabinet decided to change public hospitals into profit-making organisation, under four regional health authorities. Chapter Six reviews the lead-up to this radical change, when Cabinet swiftly terminated the control of Area Health Boards by elected members and replaced every board with appointed members. Formal community representation was altered – overnight. This sudden shift away from elected representation and towards regionalism ultimately also proved difficult, and regionalism evolved into centralised purchasing. By December 1996, many of the proposals announced in 1991 were reversed.

Chapter Seven describes how the formation of New Zealand's first coalition government, after the introduction of proportional representation at the 1996 election, provided an environment for further reform. Four purchasing agencies created under the competitive market model were merged into a single national purchaser – the Health Funding Authority. Although local representation was still off the political agenda, there was a subtle but important shift through this period towards engaging local communities in planning and decision-making, albeit within a centrally controlled infrastructure.

A change of government at the 1999 election spelled yet another round of reforms, with a new Labour Government announcing its desire to return to the health care system of district rather than centralised control. Chapter Eight details both the creation of the District Health Board (DHB) system, featuring a mix of locally elected and centrally appointed members. The chapter also discusses related policy developments through the period and provides an assessment of the structures put in place. In our concluding chapter, we review the lessons of the book and consider the future of elected boards in New Zealand.

Research sources

We close this introduction with a brief outline of sources. The main sources of data were the written records of the Department of Health and the Ministry of Health. The Ministry was established in 1993 and replaced the Department of Health. File lists were consulted for these two agencies to decide which files should be requested. At National Archives, the 'unserialised accessions' (a list of files that the Archives had not yet processed and documented) and serialised file lists were consulted. We searched lists for the Department of Health, Treasury, the Social Security Department, and Royal Commissions. Files that indicated review of policy, reform of policy, re-organisation or mentioned specific reviews identified by the case selection process were chosen. The Ministry of Health has a computerised database for all of its files. The Ministry of Health granted permission to examine the files under the Official Information Act 1982. All archival documents are cited according to the procedure used by National Archives. Page numbers are cited for reports and longer documents accessed in the archives.

Other archival documents from each reform era were examined including memos, letters, draft reports, meeting records and Cabinet papers. Parliamentary Committee reports and submissions were also examined at the Parliamentary Library. Ministerial speeches and Hansard were also consulted. Cabinet, legislative department, Hospital Boards' Association and personal file lists of politicians were also examined at National Archives. The New Zealand Medical Association granted access to their older files as well as those from the early 1970s. The main research data for political parties was derived from manifestos and internal party documents. Where possible, mass media sources were analysed. Public opinion data was analysed as well.

For the period covering the Health Funding Authority and DHB reforms, again Ministry of Health archives were searched, along with those of other central agencies, and relevant files obtained and examined. This material was supplemented with a range of interviews, including interviews with DHB chief executive officers, Ministry of Health and other officials, and observers of the reforms processes.

CHAPTER **TWO**

Cross-national models of health system governance

THE FOCUS of this book is the evolving nature and performance of local health service governance in New Zealand. However, it is useful to place these various governance arrangements and reforms over the years in comparative context. New Zealand is one of many so-called 'high-income' countries that look closely to one another for policy lessons. Comparing systems can shed light on how well arrangements have performed elsewhere and what might be learned (Blank and Burau, 2010; Gauld, 2005; Marmor et al., 2009). New Zealand's health policies have often been particularly influenced by the British National Health Service (NHS) and vice-versa. New Zealand has also sometimes been ahead of Britain in some areas. For instance, New Zealand's attempt to create a national health system came a decade before the creation of the British NHS. Moreover, in order to offset a trend of over-centralisation in planning and policy-making, the establishment of elected board members in New Zealand is something that British policy-makers have discussed as potentially desirable (Local Government Association Health Commission, 2008). Comparison shows how policies vary significantly from country to country, and a comparison with an emphasis on the historical development of policy and systems can provide insights into why such differences exist (Okma, 2010). Before exploring the New Zealand experience, this chapter distinguishes between national 'macro' and 'meso' choices related to financing and organisation, and discusses hospital organisation and governance in Australia, Britain, Canada, France, Sweden and the United States.

National or macro policy choices

In health policy we often refer to 'national' health insurance and national health services (Blank and Burau, 2010) as well as to national health systems. This generally refers to those countries where there is a government commitment to, backed by societal support for, universal health care access or insurance. Government oversees and controls the health system, intervening to ensure it caters to the population and fulfils government goals. Underpinning national systems are notions that health care access is a fundamental human right that should be available to all within a society, regardless of ability to pay.

Most systems in middle and high-income countries are broadly solidaristic in terms of striving for a degree of equity. Beyond this similarity of goals, how countries actually organise and finance care varies substantially. In some, individuals are covered by insurance; in others, they simply receive care. Bismarckian systems (after Chancellor Bismarck of Germany) are common in Europe, financing health care through social insurance premiums paid by employees, employers and general taxation. Some countries have mainly occupationally based insurance (as in Japan or France), while others allow considerable choice of insurer (such as in Germany and the Netherlands). In Australia, there is one major insurance programme (Medicare), which is financed through a mix of general taxes and the Medicare levy, with some options for individuals to purchase private health insurance. Hospitals are often either government or not-for-profit, and physicians work in private practice or on a salaried basis.

In countries with a Beveridge-style (after William Beveridge of England) 'national health service', eligibility is based on residence or citizenship rather than insurance contributions or participation. Typically, primary care is provided through independent providers in doctors' offices, but in the hospital sector government owns hospitals. Funding comes mostly from general payroll taxes and social insurance contributions, as in Britain and New Zealand, and there is universal access to services. Services are provided in kind through hospitals or, if funding is distributed to regions, sometimes allocations are determined by a population-based funding formula in which various categories that represent proxies for actual need within the community are weighted for different population groups. Formulas usually take into account age, ethnicity, rural or urban weights, as well as gender and socio-economic status. As a result, a community with higher proportions of deprived people, older people, or ethnic minorities known to be disadvantaged will receive more funds, as they are likely to have greater health care needs.

These high-income countries have health care systems that share some solidaristic goals, but it is worth contrasting these countries with one high-income outlier, the United States, which reflects the principles of individualism and a preference for the private sector to take on a larger role in financing health care. In 2009, 48 per cent of total health expenditure in the United States was government funded, in contrast with on average 80 per cent government funding across the thirty-plus OECD member countries (OECD, 2010; OECD, 2009). The majority of Americans are covered by employer-provided private health insurance, which shares some similarities with the employer-based social insurance systems. However, the American private health insurance market has historically been considerably less regulated than its equivalents in European countries, especially for those individuals not covered by employers who buy insurance independently. Under the Patient Protection and Affordable Care Act 2010, US insurers will be subject to more regulation. The government plays a substantial role in financing care for the elderly and the poor, and for government employees. It also operates an extensive health care system for veterans and military employees. However, about one in six people in the United States (close to 50 million people) lack health insurance. By law, emergency departments must treat all patients including the uninsured, the costs for whom are then recouped through higher costs for other patients and their insurers, as well as payments from states and the federal government called Disproportionate Share Hospital payments.

Meso health policy choices

Much of health policy is concerned with resolving 'meso'-level issues within these parameters of macro structures. Assuming the decisions have been made about the broader contours of insurance-based, private, or in-kind systems, there remain a number of meso-level questions that impact on regions or localities differently and may create geographically based communities of interest. Two such issues are the focus of this study: the conflict between centralisation and decentralisation of control, and the role of local communities in influencing efforts to change the spatial distribution of services or governance.

Countries frequently struggle to resolve issues around the extent to which the health care system should be centralised or decentralised

(Saltman et al., 2007), but this dynamic plays out differently in federal and national health service systems. Under federal systems, where responsibility for some funding of health care is shared between states and the federal government – such as in Canada, the United States and Australia – issues arise over who should bear the cost of expanding coverage of services and how both costs and revenues should be split. Disputes are often (but not always) influenced by challenges to and interpretations of prior agreements between states and federal governments, judicial interpretation, and constitutional convention. These are sometimes bitterly fought.

In contrast – in theory – national health systems such as in Britain, Spain, Sweden and New Zealand give the national government more latitude in dictating and changing its relationship with the periphery, especially since health care is financed mainly by national taxation. In the interests of saving money, governments may want to concentrate expensive technology or services, or focus areas of medicine in specific places. Providing a full range of medical and surgical specialties is 'not economically feasible or ecologically sensible (in terms of the numbers and distribution of people to be served) ... in small hospitals of, let us say, under 100 beds ... hence it has been necessary to develop specialisation of hospitals as well as personnel' (Roemer, 1976, p.230). Likewise, contemporary considerations of quality suggest that hospitals serving fewer than 150,000 people are 'too small to provide the necessary range of acute care services' (Healy and McKee, 2002, p.76).

Yet, even if a system is relatively centralised, governments usually encounter stiff opposition to changes in the spatial distribution or control of services. Hospitals and communities at the periphery are eager to keep their independence and local services for as long as possible. Some issues, such as which drugs should be on a pharmaceutical schedule and government-subsidised, seem more obvious candidates for centralisation. Local governance, or decentralisation of decision-making, may be more appropriate for other issues, such as where primary care or aged-care services should be located or how information technology (IT) decisions (e.g. about which software should be purchased and how systems should be configured) should be made. In New Zealand, these have traditionally been presided over locally, often because service providers identified IT needs and developed local solutions. Decentralisation has also been the result of a historic 'hands-off' approach by central government to what appears at face value to be a service-delivery issue best handled through decentralisation of decision-making (Gauld, 2004). In support of this, studies show that system-wide IT architecture with local administration is linked to lower costs, improved systems and ultimately safer and more efficient patient care (Chaudry et al., 2006). As a 'back office' function, IT illustrates how governments may approach issues, seeking to centralise those over which there may be a less evident need for local decision-making.

Hospital governance and organisation cross-nationally

Countries vary in the level of control given to hospitals at the local level, but a striking feature of the survey reported on in this chapter is that the *governance* of hospitals is likely to be a task that will continue to be decentralised and local. It reveals remarkable uniformity across both federal and national health systems, and within both public and private sectors, such as those in the United States. Hospitals require a local management structure, as well as a governing board, which usually includes people with finance, business, legal, healthcare and/or fundraising backgrounds.

While all countries have local boards, only one country has centralised hospital governance to a greater degree: Britain, which also happens to be a highly centralised state. However, surprisingly, the group of countries that have local control have little in common in other basic system features, such as whether the system is a national health service or insurance-based system. Nor do the groupings line up in terms of federal, unicameral, or other political institutional characteristics. Regional or local control of services exists in countries with a long history of local government (Sweden), as well as in countries that are supposedly highly centralised politically (France, New Zealand). Some federal (Australia, Canada, and US) systems are also decentralised.

With the exception of New Zealand, in most countries public and private hospital boards are appointed (Gauld, 2010). Two Canadian provinces had elected health boards in the 1990s, with limited success, and these were subsequently discarded. However, there is a resurgence in interest in facilitating local input into decision-making. Recent policy activity in the English NHS focused on local input (Local Government Association Health Commission, 2008), and the Scottish NHS began a pilot experiment with elected boards in two regions in 2010 (Scottish Government, 2009). The New Zealand system of elected representation, explored in this book, is instructive for its lessons on this issue.

Britain

Local government was reformed prior to the establishment of a national health service. Central government made sure it limited the ability of localities to shape hospital policy in 1946 by creating a nationalised and co-ordinated health service. Public and voluntary hospitals were reorganised into a national system of regional hierarchies with the establishment of the NHS in 1948. World War I had previously allowed Britain to reorganise the hospital sector (Webster, 1998; Tuohy, 1999). In 1948, the British government introduced the NHS that, although regionalised in many ways, has ever since been a national hierarchical structure. Only ambulance and public health services were left with local government, and municipal hospitals joined with voluntary hospitals to form 'a nationalized system' (Battistella and Chester, 1973). Indeed, the NHS today is the world's seventh-largest employer (*The Economist*, 2011), with several hundred thousand staff. Generally, voluntary hospitals and physicians feared local control of hospitals because they were concerned about its reputation for 'impecuniosity', remembering its Poor Law origins, and felt that 'democracy at the grass roots was too unpredictable and stifling to decision-making by experts' (Battistella and Chester, 1973, p.494). Nevertheless, throughout the history of the NHS, 'the balance of power between local health authorities and the centralised units of government (especially the Ministry of Health itself) has remained an area of controversy and debate' (Ruggie, 1996, p.32).

Such debates have been behind various restructurings of the NHS over the past couple of decades. For example, in the 1990s, about 300 'primary care trusts', conceptually similar to New Zealand's DHBs but with fully appointed boards, were created to plan and purchase services (called 'commissioning' in the NHS lexicon) for their respective local populations. In the 2000s, the number of primary care trusts was halved to about 150, in the belief that this would bring administrative efficiency and, with each having a larger patient population, better planning efficiency. Proposed controversial reforms introduced in 2010 could see the commissioning role performed by general practitioner groups, devolving funding and planning responsibilities directly to the primary care level, eradicating the primary care trusts and, in theory, an entire layer of administration in the process (Roland and Rosen, 2011). General practitioners would be responsible for paying hospitals directly, setting up a competition amongst hospitals for provider contracts in the process, and practitioners would have incentives to focus on keeping patients well and in the community. In turn, this could see the relevance of some hospital services called into question. Mergers are predicted for an eventual smaller number of larger, more specialised hospital facilities. However, if these reforms are implemented, general practitioner groups will need considerable support to undertake commissioning work, so it is possible that the administrative arrangements for planning and purchasing will simply be transferred to general practitioners and, therefore, become more localised. While there has been discussion in the NHS about involving the public in planning work, at present the *status quo* of appointees remains, with public input largely via 'local involvement networks', or LInKs as they are commonly referred to (Hogg, 2007).

France

The degree to which a health service is centralised is influenced by historically grounded debates about the best structure of government. For example, whereas the 'British centralized because they distrusted local government' (Ashford, 1986, p.135), the centralisation of the French state reflects historical goals of state-building and equality toward republican goals (Ashford, 1986, p.135). Hospitals were wrested from religious orders and handed over to municipalities after the French Revolution (Bridgman and Roemer, 1973). Today, although some efforts have been made in the last decade to develop more of a regional focus in health care in France, the tendency has been towards centralisation. The Schéma Régional d'Organisation Sanitaire (SROS) is used to plan the regional distribution of equipment and services. **Central government determines hospital allocations, but sickness funds distribute the money.**

France also used the war and its aftermath to impose central planning on hospital services (Bridgman, 1978), using the 1941 Hospital Act. A 1970 law established a national hospital service map (Carte Sanitaire) for planning hospital services. And, like Britain, universal health care insurance was enacted after World War II. Despite this centralisation, however, the governance of hospitals is highly localised. Local mayors are usually also presidents of hospital boards, and around one-quarter of hospital boards are elected representatives (Bridgman, 1978). A decree passed in 1997 allowed for the closure of hospitals with occupancy rates below 60 per cent, but local communities successfully opposed this and thus the decree did not lead to any widespread closure of wards or hospitals (Lancry and Sandier, 1999). Such local control of hospitals challenges the perception of France as a highly centralised country. France is considered centralised because of the overwhelming regulatory role of the central Ministry of Health in the hospital sector, and the ability of the central state to concentrate more costly services in regional centres.

Canada

The Canadian hospital system originated in a system of poor relief modelled on that of Britain. This system of charity was voluntary, until municipalities were required to assume responsibility for poor relief in the latter part of the nineteenth century by provincial governments. Provincial governments did not, however, allow municipalities to own hospitals, instead favouring subsidies to voluntary hospitals because of the religious pluralism in the east (Boychuk, 1999, p.42). Parts of Western Canada had a more rural settlement pattern that seems to have allowed municipal hospital construction in the early twentieth century (Boychuk, 1999). Western Canada looks more like Australia and New Zealand than Europe during this period. As a result, by 1957 a staggering 87 per cent of municipal hospitals were in Manitoba, Saskatchewan and Alberta (Boychuk, 1999). Nevertheless, nonsectarian and religious hospitals outnumbered these municipal hospitals. An important reason for the emphasis on voluntarism in Canada was that the religious pluralism encouraged governments to give subsidies to institutions with religious bases.

Provinces in Canada appear much more independent and less willing to seek federal solutions to their internal health care problems. Today, Canada's health care system is increasingly devolved, especially in the west. Whereas hospitals may have in the past received prospective lump sum budgets from each province, ministries of health and regional health authorities in provinces such as British Columbia, Saskatchewan and Alberta are responsible for determining the budgets for hospitals in their area (Ruggie, 1996). There are also differing models of organisation within provinces. In 2008 in Alberta, for example, several independent planning regions, each with their own appointed board, were merged into a single provincial health authority. Other provinces continue to feature multiple boards. Canada continues to explore how best to involve the public in health-care planning and decision-making, although elections are likely to remain off the agenda. As noted, in the 1990s Canada experimented with elected boards in two provinces. Following allegations that elected boards were simply set up to deal with difficult funding cuts that central authorities wished to devolve to regions, poor board performances, and an uninterested public who failed to vote in reasonable numbers (in some cases, turnout was well below 10 per cent), the model was eventually discarded (Lomas et al., 1997a; Lomas et al., 1997b; Lewis et al., 2001).

The United States
In the United States, reformers who were influenced by British policies between the two world wars proposed regionalising and planning hospital services. From the 1920s through to the 1950s, governmental and foundation-based commissions advocated regionalisation of hospitals and hospital planning. The Committee on Costs of Medical Care and the Subcommittee on Wartime Health and Education explored the deficiencies of the health service, and in 1944 the Commonwealth Fund sponsored a study of the American hospital system that also proposed regionalisation (Pearson, 1976). Immediately following the war, some other foundation and policy entrepreneurs conducted studies that advocated regionalisation, and apparently a number of states began to consider both regionalisation and planning as key goals (Pearson, 1976, p.38). President Truman also established a commission along these lines, known as the Magnuson Commission.

Efforts to make the health care system more coordinated and organised were limited. Unlike the trend in other countries of governments gradually assuming more control over hospitals, the hospital sector in the United States has remained organisationally separate. In the United States, the rise of industrial capitalism coincided with the creation of the modern independent hospital that was economically viable: most cities supported an array of autonomous hospitals. The first direct federal legislation, the Hill Burton Act of 1946, was used to stimulate hospital construction, but generally the ability of governments to fully control the hospital sector was limited. The United States' private not-for-profit and for-profit hospital sector paralleled the rise of private health insurance; this contrasts with the convergence of public financing and public hospital control seen in other countries.

Most of the efforts to develop greater regional coordination were limited in outcome, apart from state certificate-of-need programmes (which required approval of hospital facilities and, in some cases, purchases of technology). Amendments to the Social Security Act in 1972 adopted some of these policies (Pearson and Abernethy, 1980). The closest the United States ever came to a more planned health sector was the National Health

Planning and Resources Development Act of 1974, signed by President Ford (Rubel, 1976), but this ultimately failed to be implemented as planned.

Whereas governments in other countries sometimes assumed ownership of hospitals, this would have gone against the general tendency in the United States, where the government does not directly own large sectors of the economy. The underlying opposition to a generous welfare state also led to the United States' later role as funder of health care through Medicare and Medicaid in 1965. The timing of this creation meant the nation was unwilling to intervene in the delivery and ownership of medical facilities, in contrast to Britain's earlier creation of the NHS (Klarman, 1976).

There is a wide degree of variation in how hospitals are governed in the United States, depending on whether they are publicly owned. Public hospitals are sometimes – but not always – subject to oversight by locally elected officials. For example, in Los Angeles, the County Board of Supervisors is elected and supervises the public hospitals. The great majority of private and non-profit hospitals in the United States are governed by appointed board members.

The lack of direct ownership has not meant that hospitals operate without governmental control, however. There are two primary kinds of intervention. First, hospitals operate under numerous federal and state laws, including the requirement that they provide emergency care regardless of the patient's ability to pay. Non-profit hospitals have to justify their tax status by providing charity care. As well, medical record and privacy laws affect hospitals, there are limits on working hours for residents at academic medical centres and, in some states, minimum nurse–patient ratios, and standards for labour conditions and collective bargaining laws have to be observed. A second policy lever able to be applied to hospitals is federal (Medicare and Medicaid) and state (Medicaid) funding of health care. Policy-makers have drawn on their leverage as large-scale funders of hospital care to drive important hospital policy changes across all types of hospitals. For example, when Medicare required hospitals to desegregate in the 1960s, this impacted on southern states when it was applied to private hospitals (Smith, 2005). Efforts to reduce hospital costs began with Medicare payment policies – such as prospective payment using diagnostic-related groups – and moved progressively towards encouraging higher-quality facilities through reduced-payment policies (in cases of medical error) to reporting of health outcomes and quality. All of these policy initiatives change hospital behaviour; in the past, many have been adopted by private insurers.

Sweden

Sweden's hospital system is the most decentralised and the country has the longest history of explicit local government of health care. County councils assumed control of hospitals in 1863. The private health care sector is extremely small and hospitals are overwhelmingly public. Twenty county councils are responsible for almost all aspects of health care within their boundaries (Hjortsberg and Ghatnekar, 2001). County councils are elected every four years and the system of elections means voters can hold local politicians accountable for the delivery of health services (Calltorp, 1999). County councils collect local taxes to finance health services and manage local hospitals and health centres. Municipalities are responsible for long-term care. This pattern is much the same as it has been since the nineteenth century. Locally elected governments have taken on more responsibilities for health care in the last twenty to thirty years, with one of the most important reforms occurring in 1982 under the Health and Medical Services Act, and another in 1985.

Australia

Europeans settled Australia from the final decade of the eighteenth century. In the early years, hospitals in Australia's colonies were funded by local or charity-based finance plus subsidies from provincial and state governments. Settlement patterns meant that communities were very isolated from one another and initially secular voluntary associations in each community established hospitals. While the hospitals received government subsidies, they also guarded their independence (Sax, 1984, pp.22–3).

Religious orders had a strong role in the development of Australian hospitals. However, during the colonial era, and in common with Western Canada, where municipal hospital ownership was the organising structure due to the absence of a wealthy philanthropic class ready to provide finance, Australia's local hospitals relied on state government funding (Sax, 1984). They also successfully resisted nationalisation. In the oldest state, New South Wales, full public control of hospitals was proposed in 1910 but failed because hospital boards thwarted any attempts at takeover. The battle over financing hospitals began on a state level in the early twentieth century and on a national level in the 1940s, continuing until voluntary hospital insurance was introduced in 1953. Both hospitals and states in Australia appear to have needed federal support, as they were unable to survive without financial assistance. But standing in their way were physicians, who stymied a federal attempt to introduce hospital insurance in the mid-1940s. This process of controlling community-level boards appears to have come much later and was mediated by states in the 1950s (Gray, 1991).

In the 1960s, when cost inflation was beginning, federal government may have limited hospitals' ability to develop more autonomy simply by funding them inadequately. In addition, Australia's financing of hospital care through voluntary insurance began as insurance of individuals (rather than as payments made directly to hospitals) in 1953. Federal insurance benefits fell over time: 'Commonwealth policy not only undermined the states' control of hospitals but it also increased their share of financial responsibility' (Gray 1991, p.95).

The Australian states may have acted as the buffer between hospitals and the federal government, although the federal government appears to have considered national solutions to hospital financing issues as desirable. Physicians were against greater federal government financing of hospitals. Throughout the 2000s, debates about the relative roles of federal and state governments in financing hospitals have come to the fore and have been the focus of various working parties and commissions. In 2010, the federal government announced a set of health system reforms to end decades-long standoffs between the commonwealth government and states. These included centralisation of hospital funding, with all funding to come from federal government sources (Australian Government, 2010). At the same time, a series of state-funded primary care networks, known as 'Medicare Locals', was to be created to bring together various primary care practitioners to care for a geographic community (Australian Government, 2011).

Conclusion

Over time, each country develops its own particular health care and hospital system, which is shaped by intentional and unintentional constraints and laws imposed by those levels of government that are above the local level. Britain's greater control over its hospitals possibly arose from a unique set of circumstances related to World War II, followed by strenuous efforts to reorganise hospitals in 1974. But it also goes back further: English aristocrats ensured that local government was long removed from the poor law institutions that were the precursors to hospitals.

A common feature in most countries, however, is that hospitals typically are managed and controlled by a board, which guards its independence. Despite efforts to impose centralisation, communities resist changes to the spatial distribution of services by central government. Local communities and local hospitals are resilient even in countries such as France, where a centralist government finds it difficult to close, restructure, downsize or move facilities because these are electorally unpopular policies. That is not to say that the public is actively engaged in the governance of hospitals. Even in a system where they can vote, as in New Zealand, hospital politics are usually only important to the public when hospital closures, regionalisation or service changes are proposed, as we show in the chapters that follow.

The survey presented in this chapter suggests that, across all nations, hospitals may be difficult to reform. After all, hospitals are fixed capital investments with solid ties to communities (Healy and McKee, 2002, p.76). As this book argues, New Zealand boards may have been particularly resilient in their ability to retain control, even though funding increasingly shifted to the national level. From this case (and the international cases) we gain a better understanding of how local communities influence their health services, especially hospitals, through elected boards. In the next chapter, we begin the historical journey through the role and influence of New Zealand's elected boards.

CHAPTER **THREE**

The creation of universal health care, 1925 to 1960

'Cannot close hospitals.'
– John Marshall, Alexander Turnbull Library, n.d.

THE DEVELOPMENT of the Social Security Act in 1938 was a major turning point in the New Zealand health system, as it created a new system of subsidies for health care services that made health care affordable for all New Zealanders. Hospital benefits were implemented in 1939, by which hospitals were paid a daily fee for care. For hospital boards, the Act meant more funding and fewer responsibilities once the need for them to administer 'relief' (the term for social welfare) was made redundant by welfare benefits. Yet in important ways, the Social Security Act left many policy issues unresolved, and hospital boards' core governance structure remained unaltered from their nineteenth-century configuration. While the Act made hospitals more dependent on central government for funding, they continued to resist the regionalisation of hospitals.

The Labour Government's disagreements with doctors over fees left board governance unresolved. Doctors fought to maintain private funding in health care and to make government benefits means-tested. The inception of universal health care was similarly contentious in most countries (Immergut, 1992, p.67). Labour's need to resolve the remuneration of private-sector doctors may have overshadowed the need for important reforms to hospital boards in the 1930s. As a result, New Zealand established a health care system financed in two streams: one for hospital services and the other for primary care, failing to achieve a more unified national health service, as in Britain. The two sectors developed independently over the next forty years. Integrating these two systems became a focus of many reforms starting in the 1970s, which are discussed later.

This chapter tells the story behind the establishment of universally financed health care in New Zealand, beginning with a discussion of how hospital boards were key players in the debates leading up to Labour's 1938 legislation. The impetus for reform among hospital boards, doctors and taxpayers stemmed from fundamental changes in economic incentives. We also survey the late 1920s, when there were debates about the number of hospital boards and the efficiency of local administration.

The chapter skirts the edges of the better-known details of the Social Security Act and the bitter fight between doctors and the Labour Government's Cabinet. Instead, we discuss the changes for hospitals that the Social Security Act ushered in, and how the stakeholders around the hospital boards, including the farming and rural sector, perceived reform. Then we move on to show how some of the decisions of the 1930s boomeranged in the 1950s. A little more than a decade after the Social Security Act was passed, the government realised it lacked significant control over hospital boards and the hospital sector. To understand the relationship between hospital boards and central government, we must begin with the lack of resolution of this issue in the 1930s.

Strange bedfellows: doctors, farmers and hospital boards

We tend to see the creation of national health insurance as a matter of addressing the problem of inequity of access to health care. While this concern was one of many that prompted reform in New Zealand, the pressure for change was driven by three additional factors: new roles for hospitals, changing economic incentives, and new actors in the political process. Hospitals had become more attractive places to seek treatment after World War I, as they lost the stigma of their charitable origins and increased their social reputation (Fraser, 1984; Oliver, 1977).

Second, health reform emerged on the agenda in New Zealand following changes in the distribution of hospital fee payments and increases in the costs of health care in the 1920s and 1930s. Hospital boards were facing new pressures in the 1920s, caring for returned servicemen from World War I. Although their care was theoretically paid for by the Defence Department, in practice it was the boards which ended up paying for the health care of this group (Hay, 1989). Pressures for national health insurance were also partly stimulated by a Royal Commission of Inquiry that considered whether hospitals had the discretion to turn away patients. The inquiry was prompted by a complaint by a patient's father after a hospital did not admit his daughter, Miss Jessie Bryce, to the Palmerston North public hospital. Miss Bryce needed treatment for appendicitis, but the physician whom she consulted said she should seek treatment in a private hospital, saying that he believed 'public hospitals were primarily intended for patients who were not in a position to pay for private treatment' (*Evening Post*, 1924, p.5). The court decision established that public hospitals had to admit all patients and everyone had an equal right to use public hospitals in New Zealand (*Evening Post*, 1926a). While they were still able to charge differential fees for the wealthy and none for the poor, the case encouraged more people to use public hospitals (Hay, 1989, p.71; New Zealand House of Representatives, 1975).

This 1923 inquiry altered the economics of health care for the two sectors providing care, hospitals and primary care doctors, and the relative prices of each. Typically, economic historians suggest great policy and societal changes follow changes in relative prices (North, 1981), which is what happened in New Zealand health care. Doctors were already prohibited from receiving patient fees for care given in public hospitals, so upon admission to hospital patients received subsidised care from the same community doctors for far less. Doctors felt that public hospitals should have private wards, where doctors could treat their patients and charge private fees (*NZ Truth*, 1925).

Doctors were upset they were losing paying patients to public hospitals (*Evening Post*, 1926b). Hospitals were also squeezed because they faced new financial pressures when more people were admitted (*Evening Post*, 1926b). Hospital boards and ratepayers were footing the bill for free treatment and were caught between incentives to provide services for local voters and increased funding demands caused by the new admission criteria. Hospital board members were elected by citizens and therefore had to be sensitive to public opinion. Of course, public opinion was not always unified or consistent; sometimes voters pushed for lower taxes, while other citizens, who paid for some of the expenses of hospitals through local taxes, felt public hospitals should be available for free or nominal charges (Hay, 1989). For example, a Taranaki delegate to a Hospital Boards' Association (HBA) meeting in 1925 explained that a proposed fee increase would 'not suit his district, where the farmers who had paid rates for years looked upon the hospital as their own and would not allow the institution to be dominated by any other' (*Evening Post*, 1925). Board members were faced with the choice of either losing local elections or pressuring the government for more money (Hay, 1989, p.69). Rather than face losing office, board members lobbied government throughout 1929 (National Archives, 1921–41). In addition, the HBA supported compulsory insurance paid by employers as a way to reduce pressures on hospitals.

A third impetus for reform came from the new political actors entering the arena and their efforts to put the issue on the policy agenda. Starting in the 1920s, doctors, farmers and hospital boards all had reasons to push for voluntary and other forms of national health insurance, each driven by very different motivations. The framing of the issue of health care reform in the 1930s was influenced by an ongoing dialogue between doctor groups, hospital boards, farmers and local associations over fees, hospital boards and funding (see Bolitho, 1979; Hay, 1989; Lovell-Smith, 1966). Political parties also joined the debate. For example, Labour introduced health care into its election platforms in the 1920s (Hanson, 1980, p.27).

Farmers and rural residents were less prominent in this coalition, but they did play a role in putting health care reform on the policy agenda. At that time, taxation policy was very different from what it is today, with a smaller base of people paying a bigger share. The hospital boards were spending more, which put pressure on rural taxpayers because of higher taxes. Farmers considered that the tax burden was falling disproportionately on them, as opposed to town dwellers, because hospital taxes were levied on the basis of property values and farmers had large landholdings. Thus in the 1930s, farmers advocated a change in the funding of health services by which everyone would pay a 'fair contribution' and 'benefited equally' (New Zealand Medical Association, n.d.).

Government responses

This discontent prompted the government to consider introducing a scheme for national health insurance in 1925, but it made no progress (Hanson, 1980, p.27). The general trend for governments in the 1920s was towards balanced budgets (Hawke, 1984). In 1928, the Department of Health's survey of the New Zealand hospital system showed that, on average between 1915 and 1925, central government expenditure on the hospitals increased by 15.6 per cent per year (*Evening Post*, 1928). The report said that the number of hospital districts exceeded the needs of the country and the increase in the number of hospital districts was not economical. Therefore, it recommended amalgamations, although it did not say how many. And the Department's survey confirmed that rural districts were funding 60 per cent of the cost of the hospitals.

As the Depression developed, fiscal concerns came to the forefront. During 1932, hospital reform was once more on the policy agenda. This time it was sparked by a government report on reducing public expenditure, which suggested combining some hospital boards to create a Board of Hospitals responsible for managing the hospital system, which would be comprised of 16–18 hospital districts (*Guardian*, 1932j). Better transportation meant that New Zealand no longer needed forty-five hospital districts. The report recognised its position was controversial and that the recommendation '… will meet with a storm of protest', but it urged that national rather than parochial interests should prevail.

This proposal won some support from one Wellington Hospital Board member, Mr Campbell Begg, who published an article in the *Evening Post* advocating eighteen districts (*Evening Post*, 1932d). Other members of the HBA thought the idea of forming a super board was a 'most undemocratic proposal' (*Evening Post*, 1932c, p.12). Begg commented that the HBA would never recommend amalgamations because small hospitals would outvote larger hospitals on this policy issue. Parliament could not be trusted to deal with amalgamation because local '… pressure would be brought to bear which no elected minister and no government in power could withstand' (*Evening Post*, 1932d). The proposal received more enthusiastic support from the Associated Chambers of Commerce:

> It cannot be denied that the taxpayers and ratepayers have largely themselves to blame for the huge cost of the present hospital system, since by their insistence on local hospital facilities, they have more or less forced the Government into a multiplication of hospitals far beyond actual needs. Indeed, the creation of the present number of hospitals – one for almost every community – affords a classic instance of the blind parochialism of the New Zealand taxpayer, who has thereby hung a millstone of millions around his own neck (*Evening Post*, 1932e, p.12).

The government took a softer position on the issue and on 17 November 1932 introduced the Hospitals and Charitable Institutions Amendment Bill (*Evening Post*, 1932g). Introducing the Bill, the Minister of Health explained that it had the approval of the Hospital Boards' Association and that it proposed commissions led by magistrates which would investigate amalgamations of two or more hospital districts (*Evening Post*, 1932g). These would be discussed in the districts affected (*Evening Post*, 1932i). On its second reading, MPs debated the Bill for five hours, during which 'members took full opportunity to ... stress the needs of their own districts' (*Evening Post*, 1932b, p.6). One significant objection to the legislation was that it allowed Cabinet to make decisions about amalgamations through orders in council, which was an 'abrogation of Parliament's job to outside commissions' (*Evening Post*, 1932f). Likewise, Labour MP Michael Savage said that the Bill 'placed the Minister in the position of a dictator. It was flouting the Parliamentary system' (*Evening Post*, 1932h, p.9). Labour also opposed it on the grounds that it reduced government expenditure and rural districts were concerned about the effect on rural hospitals. Labour's Napier MP W.E. Barnard said 'The power is here to torpedo the hospital system.' Another called the Bill '... one of the most subtle and pernicious that has ever come before the House' (*Evening Post*, 1932h, p.12). Other MPs said the Bill was designed to benefit private practitioners and 'would play right into the hands of the British Medical Association' (*Evening Post*, 1932h, p.9). Some MPs praised the Bill, saying it would allow national interests to prevail over 'purely local considerations' (*Evening Post*, 1933, p.9). Although several MPs voted against the Bill, it passed.

Over the next few years, some ratepayers brought petitions to the government to force amalgamations, but the Bill had failed to address some of the issues boards and doctors were most concerned about. Although these two groups had disagreed at times, especially over the issue of amalgamation of hospital districts, the hospital boards and the medical profession joined forces in 1933 to form a subcommittee to examine health insurance, gaining the assistance of the Department of Health. The British Medical Association (New Zealand Branch) (BMA) doctors worked to develop a scheme for national health insurance, as they wanted means-tested subsidies that would help low-income New Zealanders pay for care. In 1935, the HBA in association with the BMA presented its plans for health care reform, which included a compulsory contributory scheme for national health insurance but with local control by hospital boards. Both groups proposed charging fees on the basis of income, a policy that was also supported by the Department of Health (Bolitho, 1979).

In August 1935, the Coalition Government started to investigate reform, proposing that local hospital boards and representatives of medical and friendly societies should administer medical services. This proposal would maintain private practice for doctors, and medical practitioners would be able to work part-time in hospitals (Hansard, 1935). This Coalition Government's scheme was not universal but relatively generous and loosely resembled the BMA/HBA plan. However, that plan was superseded by the election of the first Labour Government.

Reform on the policy agenda

Labour was elected in 1935 amid an economic depression that caused voters in many countries to reject parties that had been in power during the decline (Milne, 1966). Its popularity was also based on changing alliances and demographic shifts: voting patterns were changing in the late 1920s and 1930s, and distinct rural–urban party cleavages were developing. These divisions, between rural and urban and National and Labour, may also explain the basis of support for different health policies. Voters in large towns began to shift to Labour in 1928 and 1931 (Chapman, 1962; Chapman, 1991), with voters in the middle-income suburbs helping Labour to win in 1935 (Chapman, 1991). Likewise, farmers had become discontented with the Coalition Government and began to vote for independent candidates in the 1931 election (Wigglesworth, 1954). In 1935, they supported the Labour Party after it promised to pay guaranteed prices for primary products (Milne, 1966, p.49). Labour later lost its farmer seats in 1938 and 1943 (Chapman, 1962).

Labour promised economic restoration, direction and welfare (Chapman, 1991), as well as 'full medical, nursing, and hospital attention for invalids' and 'maintenance for invalids and their dependants during ill-health' (International Labur Office, 1936, p.236). It used the slogan 'health service as free as education' (Harris et al., 1992), and had a national strategy for increasing the accessibility of health care. Its proposals for income maintenance shifted responsibility for social welfare functions away from hospital boards to the central government. This is likely to have been welcomed by hospital boards during the early 1930s, as they were particularly challenged by the increase in expenses arising from the increased numbers of unemployed patients (*Evening Post*, 1932a).

Once in government, Labour channelled its electoral promises on health care through four *ad hoc* committees (National Archives, 1936) on national health insurance between 1936 and 1938. Minister of Finance Walter Nash instructed an officials' committee to consider 'the biggest scheme' possible

(National Archives, n.d.). He said that Cabinet would then consider the 'impracticability of certain things' (National Archives, n.d.). Because of the uncertain economy, bureaucrats were urging incremental reform that would 'fill the gaps' (National Archives, n.d.).

A group of Labour MPs surveyed a range of stakeholders – including industrial unions, employers, medical professionals, nurses' associations, masseurs, dentists, pharmacists, ambulance organisations, the HBA, counties, and municipal associations – on Labour's preferences for financing and organising health reform. In written replies and meetings with the government (National Archives, 1936–37), the responses were generally predictable, given the economic interests of the groups involved. The New Zealand Farmers' Union said that hospital charges were having an adverse impact on rural taxpayers and were affecting the price of export goods (National Archives, 1938c). It supported a restricted scheme that allowed 'freedom of choice between doctor and patient' and a role for friendly societies (National Archives, 1938c). The HBA supported changing hospital finance towards compulsory contributions and suggested that hospital boards should administer health benefits at the local level (National Archives, 1936–37). Non-government hospital providers supported a compulsory scheme but argued that the insured should be free to choose their doctor, surgeon and hospital – public or private (National Archives, 1936–37). The New Zealand Counties Association supported the establishment of government health services, but also sought changes to the use of property tax to finance hospitals. With rates, or local property taxes, being based on the capital value of properties within each hospital district, they argued that 53 per cent of the capital value of properties was in rural areas while only 41 per cent of the population lived there: hospital taxes should be based on population and not on the value of property. They also advocated local administration of the health care financed by hospital boards (National Archives, 1938b).

Despite their efforts in consulting these groups, to a large degree Labour's preferences were basically predetermined, as they had committed to a universal and free health care service prior to being elected to govern. As a result, the debates within Caucus and Cabinet over the details of the scheme did not relate so much to universality as to how to make the universal health system a reality. However, in this regard the Labour Government saw shared responsibility for hospitals continuing, with the Health Minister Peter Fraser saying in 1936 that he wanted an equitable system of financing: 'I regret that I cannot agree with the suggestion that the ratepayers should be relieved of their share of hospital costs.' He also mentioned that the new government had to consider the 'division of administrative responsibility and control in connection with hospitals and allied services' (*Evening Post* 1936, p.13).

Opposition to health care reform came mainly from doctors and their representative interest group, the BMA, which released its plan for health care reform in July 1937. This plan advocated means-tested health care, based on four income classifications, but it was widely criticised for introducing means testing and the plan was generally badly received (Hanson, 1980, ch.5). Labour's proposals had been for a broad-based programme that appealed to a range of constituencies, while the BMA proposal was less so.

Discussions through 1937 and 1938 between MPs, ministers and the medical profession failed to reach consensus (Hanson, 1980). Doctors were deeply concerned about their autonomy and income, especially if payments were to be related to the number of patients registered with each doctor (National Archives, 1937b), as the BMA was opposed to a British-style capitation model (National Archives, 1937a). However, the primary disagreement was not capitation, on which Labour eventually conceded, but means-testing. Doctors were determined that the publicly financed scheme be means-tested. To try to resolve this dispute, the Minister of Health Peter Fraser offered a fee-for-service proposal with no means test. This was rejected by the BMA: their representative Dr Jamieson replied that better use of government funds could be made. Negotiations finally broke down in February 1938 and did not resume until after the Social Security Act became law that year (Hanson, 1980).

The Social Security Act established policies that almost every interest group had been pushing for, except friendly societies. Their influence was diminished despite their significant role in providing social services. In 1935, there were 1092 lodges, with 103,612 members and an estimated 200,000 dependants (Bloomfield, 1984). Friendly societies did not actively oppose the reforms: while they had argued they should administer benefits, they did not express vociferous opposition to the Social Security Act until it was implemented. After the legislation was passed, the Grand Lodge of New Zealand wrote to the Prime Minister that the Social Security Act would be extremely harmful to friendly societies and some societies objected to the state replacing self-help measures. Perhaps friendly societies assumed the

New Zealand health insurance system would resemble the scheme adopted by the UK in 1911. For example, the Order of Foresters claimed that Labour candidates had assured friendly societies that the scheme would be similar to that in the UK, where friendly societies had prospered but were later dismayed about the possible effects of the Social Security Act on the future of friendly societies. Although they realised the implications of the New Zealand legislation were different (National Archives, 1938a), the Order of Foresters accused the Labour Government of reneging on promises made to friendly societies (National Archives, 1938a).

Other than the friendly societies, the reason there was less discord between hospital boards and the government was straightforward. Hospital boards saw hospital benefits as providing more funding, and organisations like the Counties Association had wanted to have the tax base broadened for funding hospitals. Rural groups that normally supported more conservative policies were in favour of the Social Security Act and were keen for changes to the tax rates. And while these organisations all preferred local administration, it is likely that they saw the choice of continuing to fund hospitals partly from local taxes as less desirable than nationally funded hospital benefits and maintenance of the hospital board system.

The Labour Government enacted the Social Security Act in 1938, having decided to fund the benefits under the Act equally from social security taxes and funds from the consolidated fund. The implementation of benefits occurred in stages. The breakdown in negotiations between doctors and government meant that the benefit for general practitioner services remained unimplemented until 1941, when an agreement was finally reached. As a result, the first benefit of the Social Security Act to be introduced was free treatment in psychiatric and general hospitals in 1939.

In a single legislative stroke, the Labour Government transformed the financing of hospital services in New Zealand. Ratepayers continued to contribute to the cost of hospital boards, but over time the financial provisions of the Act shifted responsibility from local ratepayers to individuals with income. Thus, ratepayers paying hospital board taxes gradually ceased to be the main source of income for hospitals, and funding was assumed by national government.

Runaway costs and hospital reform in the 1950s

From 1939, uncontroversial changes to hospital funding brought about by the Social Security Act shifted payments to hospitals. By 1943, hospitals gained their income equally from three sources: the Social Security Fund, a levy from local authorities, and the government subsidy from general taxation. Expenditure increased, which led to increases in the levies on local authorities and, as a result, 'property owners complained that they were being asked to carry an unfair burden as compared to other sections of the community' (Statistics New Zealand, 1958). During the 1940s, hospital boards found it increasingly difficult to raise funds from local sources (Heggie, 1969, pp.36–7). The government then passed legislation (the Finance Act 1946 no. 2) that limited the property taxes collected by local authorities to a halfpenny per pound of residents' rateable value. By 1951, the Social Security Fund was contributing 55 per cent of hospital costs. The Hospitals Amendment Act 1951 gradually abolished the levy paid by local authorities over the next five years (Hon. George F. Gair, 1980) and the effect of this legislation was to increase the role of general taxation in financing health care (Statistics New Zealand, 1958). By 1957, the government contribution had increased to 66 per cent (Statistics New Zealand, 1958). In April 1958, the government assumed complete financial responsibility for the public hospitals, apart from loans for major capital construction (Statistics New Zealand, 1958).

In the next section, we move to the 1940s and early 1950s, the period after the Social Security Act was implemented, to explore the formation and consequences of those policies. By 1950, the cost of supporting the social security system (which included health) was coming under attack. Government's funding of hospitals was based on a daily benefit, which provided few incentives to discourage admissions, reduce length of stay or streamline costs. Newspaper commentators criticised the high costs of the social security system and suggested that it had grown too fast and that it was not really 'free' (National Archives, 1953j). Editorials criticised the high cost of health services and expressed concern about the level of expenditure, should the economy contract (National Archives, 1950a). However, it was recognised that any party proposing a reform of the benefit system would suffer politically (National Archives, 1950b). Organised labour discussed the momentum that was gathering for severe curtailment of health services (National Archives, 1950d) and speculation was mounting over cuts to social security (National Archives, 1950c).

National assumed office in 1949 and leveraged the 1951 election (held in the midst of industrial strife) to cast Labour in an unfavourable light, after steadily gaining support in the 1940s from rural constituencies and shrewdly targeting marginal town and city districts (Chapman, 1991, p.353). The National Party won votes by promising to 'Make the pound go further' (Chapman, 1991, p.356) in a period when inflation and scarcity made voters sensitive to economic policy positions. Many of Labour's former supporters, whose economic position had improved, now shifted their support to National (Chapman, 1991, p.356). National moved closer to the political centre by accepting the welfare state, but presented itself as an alternative manager that was more efficient and less doctrinaire than Labour (Milne, 1966, p.58). The party promised voters it would prevent socialism from taking root in New Zealand and had a receptive audience for its attacks on regulations, particularly import controls, which consumers did not support (Milne, 1966, p.60). National relaxed Labour's controls on prices, capital investment, and licensing of industry, but also established agricultural producer boards (Milne, 1966, p.60).

In its 1949 manifesto, the National Party had promised to undertake a 'complete reorganisation of the entire hospital administration of New Zealand ... based on regional control and decentralisation' (Dow, 1995, p.173). The party platform supported regionalisation as a step towards better services and facilities and greater efficiency at less cost (Marshall, 1983). While National said it was concerned about escalating spending on social security (including health), it also believed that more hospital beds were needed in some areas. One of the principal differences between Labour and National was the latter's more favourable view of private providers. The National Government established loans for private hospital construction in 1952 and extended these in 1954 (Department of Health, 1969).

The context throughout the 1950s was clearly one of fiscal conservatism and rising expenditure on health care. Hospital boards had also started to make greater demands for buildings, equipment and additional staff and had a different outlook towards the financing of hospitals (Hon. George F. Gair, 1980). The amendment of the Social Security Act in 1951 gave ministers as well as the Department of Health a greater incentive, and justification, for being more closely involved in scrutinising hospital board activities.

The first push for regionalisation

The National Government was determined to reorganise hospitals. The government had successfully joined six hospital boards and formed a single district in one area of New Zealand, thus reducing the number of hospital boards to thirty-seven in 1950 (Department of Health, 1969). In 1952,

Health Minister John Marshall worked with the Department of Health to extend this plan to other boards. He argued that health care reform was necessary, given changes in transportation and the need to control government expenditure. He wanted to bring hospitals up to date and develop regional hospitals, to avoid duplication of equipment and services. Marshall observed that, whereas local financing had once encouraged excessive thrift, by the early 1950s the problem had become excessive expenditure by hospital boards. However, Marshall's own notes suggest that he also recognised the political obstacles to reform, noting, 'Cannot close hospitals' (Alexander Turnbull Library, n.d.).

John Marshall and the Department of Health both supported the creation of a Royal Commission as a way of resolving the issue. The Department shared Marshall's views on hospital rationalisation and representation, and the desirability of reducing the number of hospital boards (Alexander Turnbull Library, 1952a). It had drafted the 'Hospital Consolidation Bill' proposing rationalisation in 1952, but deferred its introduction because it would be involved in the Commission (Alexander Turnbull Library, 1952b).

Marshall announced the plans for reorganisation at a HBA meeting, which immediately passed a resolution opposing the establishment of the Commission (Marshall, 1983). The Commission was asked to make recommendations to the government on 'the reform of the present hospital system' (Consultative Committee on Hospital Reform, 1953), and its official title was the Consultative Committee on Hospital Reform, but it was also commonly known as the Barrowclough Commission (after the Chairman, H.E. Barrowclough). It was charged with examining the constitution, functions, powers and duties of hospital boards, the number of hospital districts, and the possibility of establishing regional base hospitals. The government firmly indicated its desire to restructure the hospital system and asked for submissions from the public.

The Barrowclough Commission held hearings all over New Zealand and became a focal point for those unhappy with the spectrum of hospital reform and closures. At the same time, some supported change. In Dunedin, the Commission heard from the Otago Hospital Board, which said it supported the plan and presented a proposal for four base hospitals in New Zealand, with two on each island. Otago medical staff suggested that local hospital boards should remain and function as management committees (National Archives, 1953g). The New Zealand Registered Nurses'

Association supported the amalgamation of hospitals with fewer than fifty occupied beds. The British Medical Association (New Zealand Branch) supported the reduction of hospital districts and agreed that base hospitals should be linked to smaller hospitals (National Archives, 1953e).

People representing hospitals and townships that could lose their hospital board strongly opposed any changes. Boards such as Hawera and Dannevirke presented optimistic views of the existing arrangements and argued that no changes should be made from present democratic local control and representation (National Archives, 1953f). Thames Hospital argued the need for close proximity of services for maternity patients (National Archives, 1953h). In the south, a variety of organisations opposed change, from farmers, borough councils, ratepayers to business (National Archives, 1953i).[1] On the West Coast, mayors, local officials and business associations also pleaded for local control and representation to be retained by towns, and community groups rallied in support of their hospitals (National Archives, 1953d).[2] Individuals in these communities wrote letters to the commission and individuals mentioned the capital funding their communities had given hospitals over the years. One council wrote that local taxpayers had worked hard to establish their local hospital and those taxpayers and residents 'had always taken a keen personal interest in the welfare and administration of their own particular local institution' (National Archives, 1953a).

In it submission at the Wellington hearings, the Department of Health presented a very different profile of hospitals and hospital boards, describing the existing hospital system as anachronistic, and citing the number of times rationalisation had failed in the late nineteenth century. The Department advocated a reduction in hospital boards, better control of finance, and a system of regional base hospitals. It saw the importance of

---

1. The South Otago Hospital Board mentioned that locals wanted to retain control of the hospital and was supported by local groups and local government. An array of organisations, from the Bruce County Council, the Balclutha Borough Council, the Clutha Lodge IOOF, the Kaitangata Borough Council, the Federated Farmers (Balclutha Branch), the Milton Borough Council, the Owaka Ratepayers Association, the Balclutha Businessmen's Association to the Clutha County Council, endorsed the existing system of local control (see National Archives 1953d).
2. On the West Coast, the Women's Institutes of Nokihinui, Hector-Ngakawau, the Buller County Council and County Residents, the Buller Progress League (an organisation of business people and local bodies), the Denniston, Millerton, Seddonville and Stockton Colliery and Karamea Medical Associations, representing 1100 members of the mining farming and saw-milling fraternity of the Buller District, also presented evidence (see National Archives 1953b).

having hospitals locally controlled by a community of interest that could be held accountable to the public, but argued that a small population made it impracticable to reconcile local accountability with efficiency (National Archives, 1953c). The Department also said that some communities were beginning to realise that regional hospitals provided a wider range of services than local hospitals and that this had created 'a tacit understanding' that some hospitals were in effect base hospitals for small adjacent hospital districts (National Archives, 1953b).

After hearing evidence, the Barrowclough Commission reported its findings (Consultative Committee on Hospital Reform, 1953). The Commission members agreed with the Department of Health that hospitals were organised on the basis of nineteenth-century patterns. They called small, localised hospitals 'historical relics' and pointed out that rationalisation of hospital boards had long been on the agenda. Hospitals were funded by central government but administered at the local level. Board members had few incentives to conserve resources, since financing was not raised locally. Some boards had admitted to the Commission that after government began to pay a larger share, their requests for funding had become more liberal. The commission presented evidence that some hospital boards spent twice as much as others *per capita*.

The Barrowclough Commission recommended that responsibility for providing health services should be transferred from hospital boards to the Minister of Health and that five regional authorities be established to coordinate, direct and control the activities of hospital boards, along the lines of the British National Health Service Act. The number of boards would be reduced to a total of twenty-three, with each regional authority retaining its 'base' board. Regional authorities were to be staffed by appointed members. Base or metropolitan boards were to have four appointed members added to a predominance of members elected on a geographical basis; all other boards were to remain wholly elective.

Surprisingly, only the first recommendation of the commission was embodied in the Hospitals Act of 1957 (Department of Health, 1969), which set·out new relationships (Heggie, 1969, pp.36–7). But the Act stayed away from prescribing specific reductions in boards. The Act had the potential to change the structure of health services. Under the new law, the Minister of Health, on behalf of the government, was given responsibility for ensuring the provision by hospital boards of hospital and associated services, and the government assumed complete financial responsibility for hospitals. The Minister was given wide powers of direction and regulation to ensure the establishment of a comprehensive and integrated new hospital service for the whole country (Statistics New Zealand, 1968). The Minister of Health could intervene in decisions on loans, capital expenditure, staff appointments and closure of institutions or restriction of services, with the agreement of the Hospitals Advisory Council (Statistics New Zealand, 1958).

The Hospitals Act 1957 had considerable potential but failed to alter significantly the governance structures of hospitals. Implementation of the Act could have brought about reorganisation of the entire hospital sector. Instead, 'the new Hospitals Act simply subjected the hospital boards to further restraint' (Department of Health, 1975, p.64). The Act provided for the establishment of the Hospitals Advisory Council, comprising three departmental members (Health, Treasury and Works) and three hospital board members. The rules of the council required a two-thirds majority (Statistics New Zealand, 1958) and it was the intention of the National Government that the Council would 'play an important advisory and leadership role in hospital services' (Department of Health, 1975, p.65). Instead, its main use was to advise the Minister on issues of contention between the Department of Health and local interests (Department of Health, 1975). Furthermore, the Commission's recommendation for regional health authorities was not implemented. The Commission's third recommendation – of reducing the number of hospital boards from thirty-seven to twenty-three – also made no progress until the late 1960s, when the issue returned to the policy agenda. In 1968, some hospital boards amalgamated and the total number of boards shrank from thirty-seven to thirty-one.

Conclusion

The Social Security Act is widely considered to be the legislation that underpins the health service. Yet, when New Zealand's system of payments for hospital services made to highly localised and powerful boards is compared with Britain's more unified National Health Service, this assumption is tested. New Zealand's reform introduced not so much a *health service* as a system of payment for *health services*. This difference is partly explained by Labour's focus on creating a national funding system for primary care, which overshadowed the need for important reforms to hospital boards in the 1930s. But the debates and battles of the late 1920s also made it clear that this was not an issue that would win friends for Labour.

By the 1950s, some of the same issues were as challenging for policy-makers as they had been in the 1920s. Two parallel payment systems developed, with different accountability structures. The Barrowclough Commission was supposed to provide the platform for regionalisation. Whereas professional resistance had curtailed Labour's ambitious plans in primary care, National's new plans for the health service in the 1950s suffered a different fate. Local hospital boards, and communities themselves, rallied to oppose the government. The public expressed alarm at the plans to reduce boards' powers and autonomy (Department of Health, 1975). Hospital boards successfully protested the expansion of state control in much the same way that doctors did in the late 1930s. Hospital boards prevented the government from reshaping the hospital sector through their veto over hospital policy.

Hospital boards increased their financial dependence on central government in 1938 and again in the early 1950s. However, hospital boards strongly resisted government proposals that local boards yield more control over hospital policy in exchange for increased funding. The Barrowclough Commission raised the issue of the lack of accountability in hospitals but government found itself unable to make large-scale policy changes to the hospital sector due to strong local pressure throughout New Zealand. By 1960, central government had expanded its bureaucratic capacity towards more emphasis on health policy-making.

The Barrowclough Commission on Hospital Reform was critical in that it established a principle of regionalisation that stayed on the agenda for the remainder of the twentieth century. The Commission may also have had the unintended effect of showing hospital boards that they had the power to influence policy and may, therefore, have set a precedent for opposition to future government reform proposals.

CHAPTER **FOUR**

Rational planning meets democratic forces

B Y THE late 1960s and during the 1970s, the government faced intense pressure to reform the hospital sector. Waiting lists rose and the Naitonal Government helped the private sector to expand so that it could meet demand. In 1971, it established the Royal Commission on Hospital and Related Services to consider health care reform. When Labour won the next election, it abolished the Commission in 1972 and initiated its own study. Other chapters show how all efforts at hospital reform were flavoured by larger economic and social events, as well as fashions in policy-making. For example, the Depression in the 1930s prompted universalism, while the 1980s and 1990s was an era when policy-makers redefined the relationship between markets and government.

The 1970s approach to hospital reform was influenced by two factors: (1) the economic context and changing ideas about the economy, government and public policy, and (2) new ideas and critiques of medical care itself. These factors acted as kindling for the newly energised Labour Party. The economic context profoundly influenced the choices available to New Zealand. Commodity prices fell and the country experienced unfavourable terms of trade. As national income declined in the late 1960s, New Zealand developed a penchant for so-called 'rational planning' in all aspects of public policy. In some ways, this reflected long-standing Vogelian big-government ideas rather than a new development. This was the era during which New Zealand began forming think-tanks such as the Planning Council (later disbanded in the spending cuts of the 1990s). Health care was just one of many areas up for review, and the government completed comprehensive investigations of many policy areas in the late 1960s. There was faith in the potential for control and scientific organisation in the health sector. Similar ideas were expounded in other countries, even in the United States, although there the trend was short lived in health. A second factor was contemporary leftist critiques: Ivan Illich decried the medicalisation of society in 1975, Thomas Szasz critiqued traditional treatment methods for mental illness, Eliot Freidson questioned the elevated professional authority of doctors (Freidson, 1970) and Arnold Relman coined the term 'medical-industrial complex' (Relman, 1980). Feminists argued that health care should be more responsive to consumers and that providers should be more aware of women's needs (Coney, 1993). These larger trends set the scene for a reconsideration of the role of hospitals, a call for more community-based care, and raised the first consumer-oriented challenge to the way health services were organised.

Reform in the 1970s

Initially in the late 1960s, the Department of Health, doctors and (to a lesser extent) the National Party defined the agenda for reform. National asked the Minister of Health to reform hospitals, suggesting that the hospital board system was a carry-over from the days of local funding (National Archives, 1969a). National's manifesto in the 1969 election promised to transfer all state-financed hospitals to hospital boards and to merge hospital districts (New Zealand National Party, 1969).

Civil servants in the Department of Health were the most instrumental in this process and may have had the advantage of being insulated from direct electoral consequences. The state can formulate and pursue goals with considerable autonomy from social groups or interests (Skocpol, 1985). In the 1960s, the Department of Health expanded its role in health policy, planning and research, and wanted to reduce its non-policy and operational activities (National Archives, 1969–70). The Department firmly committed itself to the hospital reform policy in a 1969 report on the hospital system (Department of Health, 1969). Officials were influenced by regionalisation in Britain and argued that a similar approach would break the stranglehold of the hospital boards and thus encourage the consumer voice (National Archives, 1969–70). The Department argued that boards could be rationalised and reconstituted as health boards (Dixon, 1969) and advocated some transfer of responsibilities to the hospital boards. In practice, the Department might have proved less willing to surrender its jurisdiction in the health arena to the local level than it claimed.

A Department of Health survey of hospital services in 1969 provided the empirical data for subsequent proposals. The survey counted 31 hospital boards responsible for 197 hospitals, which included 75 general hospitals (including three that also contained senior-citizen institutions), 81 maternity hospitals, 20 special hospitals and 20 senior-citizen institutions (Department of Health, 1969, p.23). Forty-one per cent of all public hospitals were maternity hospitals. General hospitals accounted for 38 per cent of public hospitals. In the private sector, 151 private hospitals also provided 3495 beds, or around 16 per cent of all hospital beds in New Zealand.

Clear disparities in beds between hospital boards were evident in the late 1960s. Many areas of the country that were less populated retained more hospital beds *per capita* than areas where the population was growing. While Auckland, the largest city in New Zealand, had 3.6 general hospital beds per 1000 people, some less populated areas of New Zealand had 9.2 hospital beds per 1000 people. Eleven hospital boards existed to serve less than 1 per cent of the population.

At first, in 1970, the government asked nine hospital boards to amalgamate, but only one agreed (Department of Health, 1969, p.69). The Department of Health succeeded in merging eight of the tiniest hospital boards in 1969, 1972 and 1975 and closed six hospitals in 1969. The Department then closed only one in 1972 and one in 1975.

Doctors comprised the second main group promoting health care reform, beginning their advocacy in 1967 (Editorial New Zealand Medical Journal, 1968a). The Medical Association of New Zealand (MANZ) published its own comments on health care reform, suggesting private health insurance and recommending decentralisation of medical decision-making to local levels (New Zealand Medical Journal, 1968b). The MANZ wanted control of health services to be taken away from ratepayers and local authorities and placed in the hands of six or fewer district bodies (National Archives, 1971–73). A breakaway group of doctors, the New Zealand Medical Association,[1] advocated state control of the health service by an autonomous body or corporation with government representation (National Archives, 1973).

---

1. The MANZ later took this name as its own after the NZMA dissipated in 1974.

Table 3. Numbers of general hospital beds relative to population, by board, 1969

Source: Department of Health, 1969

Hospital board	General hospital beds per 1000 population
Dannevirke	9.2
South Otago	8.5
Thames	8.4
Wairoa	8.3
Opotiki	7.8
Westland/West Coast	7.7
Taumarunui	7.3
Cook	6.9
South Canterbury	6.9
Maniototo	6.7
Marlborough	6.7
Vincent	6.7
Waipawa	6.4
Northland	6.3
Hawkes Bay	6
Waitaki	6
Wanganui	5.9
Otago	5.8
Palmerston North	5.6
Waiapu	5.6
Tauranga	5.5
Ashburton	5.3
Taranaki	5.1
Southland	5
Wellington	5
Wairarapa	4.4
Bay of Plenty	4.3
Waikato	4.3
Nelson	4.1
North Canterbury	4
Auckland	3.6
Mean	6.1
Weighted mean	4.9

The National Government established the Royal Commission on Social Security,[2] which could have resulted in a fundamental review of the health policies of 1938; however, at the request of Cabinet, hospital benefits were left out of the terms of reference (National Archives, 1969b). The Government thinking was that a separate inquiry was necessary for hospitals. Once again, as in the 1930s, a widespread review of social policies left out the question of how hospitals and hospital services fit into the welfare state. Cabinet seemed hesitant about engaging in a full reform process and government was unsure whether it should establish a mental health inquiry or an investigation of the whole health care system. As often occurs in policy-making, reform moved on to the policy agenda when prompted by a 'focusing event' (Kingdon, 1995), that began as a dispute at a psychiatric hospital. At issue were changing employment conditions, caused by a transfer of responsibility for mental health institutions from the Department of Health to hospital boards (Medical Association of New Zealand, 1971). By October 1971, the Prime Minister announced that Government had made a firm decision: the proposed inquiry would cover the entire field of hospital services. In 1972, the National Government established the Royal Commission on Hospital and Related Services. The composition of the inquiry represented a mixture of business figures, medical professionals, and laypersons.[33] The Royal Commission intended to fundamentally examine the health care system but, as the discussion below shows, its life was brief and its terms of reference narrower than other reform episodes. This turned out to be the shortest and most insignificant of the reform episodes surveyed in this book: the Commission lasted only until early 1973 (National Archives, 1973a).

To a great extent, the issue that prompted reform actually became its focus: despite its broad mandate, the Royal Commission focused more on the issue of mental health services than on the broader issue of health care reform. Much of the Commission's submissions were concerned with the payment and conditions of psychiatric nurses and the system of mental health administration in New Zealand (See National Archives, 1972b, 1973). A few submissions did highlight the problems in the sector as a

---

2. The Commission concerned itself mainly with income support aspects of the social security system and, despite the economic conditions, recommended that social benefits should be expanded.
3. The chairman of the Commission was Charles Pierrepont Hutchinson, who was also the chairman of the Oakley Hospital Inquiry. Other members of the Commission were James Richard Cropper, Wilton Ernest Henley, John Turnbull, and Iona Williams.

whole (National Archives, 1972a). One submission painted a portrait of health services influenced by the previous system of local financing, and proposed board rationalisation and the creation of a national commission.

The Labour Government ultimately took up these ideas on health care organisation between 1972 and 1975, but Labour disbanded the Royal Commission on 9 March 1973 (National Archives). The Commission issued three reports, mainly on mental health issues related to pay rates for nurses and services for mentally handicapped patients. The first report was tabled in Parliament on 6 March 1973 (Hansard, 1973). Once National had been voted out of office, the work of the Commission was superseded. Labour said it feared that the Royal Commission would take too long to report and take action, believing that results were required quickly (National Archives, 1973b). For once, the health reform process was torpedoed by government, rather than by hospital boards.

Efforts at regionalisation between 1972–84

During the period 1972 to 1984 policy-makers continued to attempt the re-organisation of hospital governance and regionalisation of hospital services. In summary, and further discussed in the sections that follow, the Labour Government published a White Paper on Health Services in 1974, but this White Paper was scuttled by a wide array of interest groups. Then Labour lost the election in 1975. The new National Government appointed a Special Advisory Committee on Health Services Organisation (SACHSO), which reinvented elements of Labour's plans of 1975, repackaged them, and worked to gain acceptance from health interest groups, particularly hospital boards. This period was a race with many false starts and no finishing line in sight (West, 1981). Prior to Labour's attempts, the earlier National Government had been making some progress on amalgamating some of the smaller hospital boards. After the White Paper, hospital board numbers stayed static for fifteen years, since no government wanted to risk the political costs of closing hospitals or merging boards.

Labour's caucus committee on health and the 'White Paper'

Labour defeated National in the 1972 election. Labour won 55 seats, or 63 per cent of all seats in Parliament, but only 48 per cent of the votes (Harris et al., 1992). Labour was successful in provincial cities and in the South Island because it promised regional development to the rural regions (Eagles and

James, 1973). Labour also found support among liberal, young, university-educated city-dwellers opposed to the Vietnam War. Voters concerned with environmental and social issues transformed the Labour Party, following trends in other social democratic parties in Western democracies. In the 1969 election, candidates from professional backgrounds featured in the candidate line-up, and one faction proposed removing the word 'labour' from its party name because of the union connotations (Templeton and Eunson, 1969).

After being in opposition for many years, Labour entered office with strong reformist orientations. Labour's election manifesto promised to substantially reform health care. The Prime Minister noted that voters in the 1972 election were concerned about the deterioration in health services (Kirk, 1975). On that score, the most visible indicator of the health care system's performance was lengthening waiting lists. During Labour's term, in 1974, 31,840 people were waiting for surgery and 65 per cent had been waiting more than three months (some over two years) (National Archives, 1974).[4]

Labour formed a Caucus Committee on Health to examine options for reform. Over the next two years, between 1972 and 1974, officials from the Department of Health and the Committee drafted a reform plan with little participation from interest groups or the public. The Department of Health was an important influence in this health reform proposal and its submissions were well represented in the final document. The Department was in favour of regional organisations that would be responsible for a whole range of health services, including preventive, community, environmental and treatment services (National Archives, 1973–77).

In December 1974, the Labour Government released *A Health Service for New Zealand* (also known as the 'White Paper'). The underlying ethos of the White Paper reflected the growing awareness of the possible limits of medical care services to improve health alone. But it also reflected distinctly Labour concerns, as well as its electoral base in urban and lower-income communities. The problems, interpreted by Labour, were inequality and the health needs of low-income individuals, threats to universalism, and there was a concern about the growing role of the private sector in health care in New Zealand.

According to the White Paper, the policies of 1938 had failed in recent

---

4. Calculated from data on waiting lists.

years to improve health or redistribute health care resources. The Minister of Health, Tom McGuigan, pointed out that New Zealand's mortality indicators had worsened relative to other countries, that the distribution of primary care doctors was unequal, and that low socio-economic status areas were receiving fewer services and less government financing than wealthy areas. The Minister of Health proclaimed he wanted to de-emphasise traditional aspects of medical care. He stressed the government's desire to consider health care more broadly, beyond 'doctors, nurses and hospitals'. McGuigan criticised the lack of attention to public health compared to the 'gadgetry of medical technology housed in expensive hospitals' (National Archives, n.d.).

Labour's proposals reflected earlier Health Department research (Department of Health, 1969) and drew on the Barrowclough Commission (see previous chapter) explicitly. The White Paper traced the historical origins of hospital policy from the failure of capitation in the 1930s to the modern problems of the 1970s. Fundamentally, the framing of the problems in New Zealand at the time reflected Labour's more urban base and its concerns for residents of cities, including Auckland, rather than the southern rural electorates. The Department of Health had consistently described hospitals as archaic in their administration. In its deputation to the Caucus Committee, the Department described how the system of local representation had 'perpetuated parochialism' and described it as outmoded (National Archives, 1973c). In the 1930s, the Nash/Fraser leadership combination had yielded a plan for financing health care based on values of solidarity. In the 1970s, Labour's plan was to use a more rationalised, scientific management approach that drew more heavily on bureaucratic than on political norms. The White Paper drew on Health Department ideas when it proposed an elaborate system of administration, illustrated in a complex organisational chart. The Department recommended fourteen regions to be financed on a programme basis (e.g. hospital, home help, and rehabilitation), with funding weighted by age, race or economic status (National Archives, 1973d).

Under the White Paper proposals, the Minister of Health was to have greater control over the services provided by the hospital boards. Regional health authorities would be compelled to meet requirements posed by the Minister of Health. The government claimed to want to link the administration of the health service at the local level to national plans and regional health authorities. Central advice and control over finances would ensure value for money. Regional health authorities were to be responsible for regional planning of services. A New Zealand Health Authority would replace the Department of Health. In the future, hospitals were to be components in a system where health services would be planned regionally and rationally (Department of Health, 1975). Provider organisations, including primary care, hospitals and community services, would be managed by the multiple administrative agencies under the guidance of the Minister of Health. The paper also suggested that health districts should be re-organised and reduced in number (Department of Health, 1975, p.83).

The government described the various options for primary care, including a contracting system, a salary service establishing a state-funded fee without patient charges, completely privatising general practice services, and retention of the existing arrangements. While the White Paper did not establish a preferred alternative (the report said discussion was desirable), the government subtly indicated that it preferred a service based on contracts between the government and primary care doctors.[5]

As is often the case, the political response to these policy proposals sealed their fate. Reformers made an error in formulating these proposals without interest group participation. The deliberate avoidance of consultation between government and interest groups during the formulation of the White Paper was probably related to the ghosts of the 1930s. If constant references to this period in discussions on health care are any indication, the struggle between the government and doctors and the final acquiescence to the medical profession in the 1930s haunted many members of the Labour Government. In contrast to the 1930s, when plans were discussed relatively openly with the medical profession, the early 1970s represented a different model of elite negotiation between bureaucrats and ministers. The consequence, as in the 1990s, was that groups resented the government's lack of consultation over the health proposals. The White Paper reform plan envisioned a very large role for the state, which not only alienated professionals but also made enemies in the voluntary and private sectors. Again, this partly reflected Labour's greater faith in government and its urban base of support.

---

5. The White Paper was extremely critical of the fee-for-service primary care system that was described in an earlier chapter. Antipathy toward this policy may have reflected Labour-inspired bitterness from the late 1930s.

Interest group reaction

The reaction of interest groups to Labour's proposals was largely negative. Many joined forces to oppose the reform plan. The White Paper had few supporters and many opponents, partly because it proposed such sweeping reform, and extensive government regulation of the health sector. The proposal provided few benefits for the voluntary or private sector, so these groups stood alongside unionised and professional groups in opposing the plans. Their concerted effort at publicly criticising the reform plan scuttled the Labour Government's hopes of implementing change before 1978.

The medical profession is perhaps remembered for making the most trenchant critique. Doctors did lead the charge against Labour's plans. However, as this chapter shows, other groups were somewhat sympathetic to their claims. The medical profession and the hospital boards felt alienated, and even groups who supported some of the ideas of the White Paper were critical (Jack and Robb, 1977). The Medical Association of New Zealand (MANZ),[6] which represented doctors, foreshadowed political patronage and extensive bureaucratic control of the health sector by a government 'obsessed with foisting on New Zealand a top-heavy bureaucracy' (New Zealand Medical Association). The MANZ believed all professions would suffer, describing the plan as 'a threat to all free entrepreneurs'. The MANZ argued for continued fee-for-service remuneration and increased payment levels for many benefits, and incentives for under-doctored areas to attract doctors.

As in the 1930s, doctors received support from the opposition. The MANZ worked with the National Party and was consulted on party policy. In addition to meeting with the party, doctors also apparently gave substantial donations to the National Party (MANZ, 1975) (Bassett, 1976). The Leader of the Opposition asked the MANZ to examine their draft health policy in 1975 and suggested that National was interested in meeting with the Medical Association (Bassett, 1976). National promised in one draft of its 1975 manifesto to make primary care doctors the core element in the health system. It also promised assistance for doctors to hire practice nurses and loans for establishing medical practices and building upgrades. As well, National promised to allow primary care doctors to care for their own patients in hospital, and to offer incentives to encourage doctors to move to under-doctored areas. Finally, National promised to offer travel subsidies to New Zealand doctors abroad who wished to return home, together

---

6. This was the same organisation that opposed Labour in the 1930s but now the organisation was autonomous from the British Medical Association.

with attractive salaries on a full- or part-time basis in hospital service or community care.

The MANZ encouraged other groups to publicly criticise the White Paper (MANZ, 1975), and it coordinated action against it with help from public relations consultants (Bassett, 1976). The MANZ also organised a meeting of interest groups in May 1975 (New Zealand Medical Association, 1975d); the interest groups[7] questioned the need for the large-scale reforms suggested in the White Paper and proposed a review with public consultation. Generally, they agreed that the government had failed to provide compelling evidence or systematic analysis of the shortcomings of the existing system (New Zealand Medical Association, c. 1975) and had embarked on reform in haste. Groups were very uncertain that the promised benefits of the reform would ever materialise.

Organisations representing medical specialists questioned whether people were significantly dissatisfied with the health care system, and argued that standards would not be improved under the White Paper. One medical specialist group described the faith in administrative control as 'naïve' and suggested serious problems were treated superficially (New Zealand Medical Association, 1975c). General practitioners proposed keeping the fee-for-service system (New Zealand Medical Association, 1975a). Nurses were less critical of the White Paper than other groups (New Zealand Medical Association, 1975b). Nurses had been more sympathetic to the aims of Labour Governments historically and, as a major unionised group, had an entrée into the Labour Party. Despite their muted criticisms when compared to their medical colleagues, they were upset about the lack of plans for nursing education. Hospital physiotherapists were more pessimistic. The Hospital Boards' Association posed incremental reform as the answer. The Plunket Society, a non-profit society organised to improve the health of infants and young children, commented that it was concerned about the lack of voluntary participation in preventive medicine.

Private health insurers were extremely critical of the White Paper and disagreed that the private health sector was crowding out the public.

---

7. General Practitioner Society; Medical Association of New Zealand; Medical Officers of Schools Association; Municipal Association of New Zealand Inc.; National Society on Alcoholism and Drug Dependence New Zealand Inc.; New Zealand Dental Association Inc.; New Zealand Institute of Medical Laboratory Technology Inc.; New Zealand Private Hospital Association; New Zealand Society of Chiropodists Inc.; New Zealand Society of Physiotherapists Inc.; New Zealand Society of Radiographers Inc.; New Zealand State Dental Nurses Institute; The Plunket Society; Southern Cross Medical Care Society; Wellington and Hutt Valley Nurses Bureau.

Organisations representing consumers also opposed the plans. The National Council of Women complained about the lack of time doctors were able to devote to patients and the delays in gaining hospital admission. Only a minority of the Council's membership wanted a completely free service. Instead, the Council advocated nominal fees, with some exceptions for young children, the elderly, the handicapped and those in hardship, and argued that private services should continue to provide choice (New Zealand Medical Association, 1975a). The New Zealand Public Health Association criticised the cost of the proposals, the lack of detail in the document, and suggested that the existing system of public and private provision should be continued. A group of citizens urged the government to 'halt its hasty "rash" of blind bureaucratic socialistic legislation' (New Zealand Medical Association, 1975a).

Despite the negative reaction, the White Paper was important. In the long run, it was useful because it stimulated public debate on health care services (Brunton, 1983). The attempted policy reform between 1972 and 1975 had an agenda-setting influence, and some of the ideas were translated into future reform plans. However, in the short term, the government had created a reform plan that only served to alienate every single health interest group.

Given the framing of the proposals by interest groups, it is not surprising that Labour's plan was also poorly perceived in the public arena. Press coverage of the White Paper was not sympathetic. Politicians under-estimated the public readiness for reform and managed the political conflict over the White Paper poorly. The document was inaccessible and difficult for consumers to comprehend (Brunton, 1983), although this seems to be a feature of health care reform proposals worldwide and in different periods. An analysis of the political acceptability of the plan in November 1975 (National Archives, 1976d) noted widespread opposition. The public associated the plan with bureaucracy, especially the Department of Health, but they had little idea of what the Department did. In response, the Department of Health proposed expanding its public relations capacity in 1976, to encourage contact with interest groups and 'special publics', as well as monitor press coverage in district offices (National Archives, 1976a). The government as a whole, however, did not work hard to promote the policies proposed in the White Paper. Advisers suggested that if Labour was to be re-elected it should vigorously seek public support and that the Government should seek the co-operation of interest groups to encourage implementation of the White Paper. National ended up taking this advice when it was elected in 1975.

Meanwhile the White Paper called for submissions and, by October 1975, 394 submissions had been received on reorganisation. Consultative groups were then established (National Archives). In their submissions to these, numerous groups requested more public involvement in the development of health care services (National Archives, 1976d). However, Labour was voted out of office at the end of 1975. Thus, Labour's plan was a casualty of the 1975 election, but health did not necessarily cause Labour to lose the election. The economy was the leading issue for voters (9.3 per cent), followed by the issue of retirement pensions (6.3 per cent) (Social Science Data Archives, 1975). Fifty per cent of voters considered the Labour Government had performed a fair job (Social Science Data Archives, 1975).

National capitalises on Labour's failure

National fought the 1975 election on a platform against centralisation and big government, while simultaneously also promising to expand the welfare state. National won fifty-five out of eighty-seven seats in Parliament (Harris et al., 1992). Labour's loss in 1975 provided National with a fresh opportunity for reform. The next era of health care reform in the late 1970s and early 1980s marked a distinct break from previous efforts, in reaction to the White Paper of 1974–5 (Brunton, 1983). According to one former government official, the White Paper 'cast a shadow on all future plans' (Martin, 1997). National wanted its policies to be completely disassociated from Labour's plan once it was in office.

Labour's failure to reform health had generated a process of political learning amongst both politicians and bureaucrats. Labour's defeat meant that 'the conventional wisdom in political circles for the next decade was that health service reorganisation was a heavy electoral liability' (Martin, 1991, p.279). Bureaucrats stated that the political sensitivity of hospital board boundaries would preclude any imposed alteration of these boundaries in the foreseeable future (National Archives, 1978). In contrast to Labour, National did not see either the possibility or the necessity of rapid results and adopted a conservative approach designed to alienate as few interest groups as possible. As a result, board numbers stayed static for the next fifteen years and few changes were initiated (Department of Health: Division of Hospitals, 1967–84).

National exploited Labour's failed attempt at health care reform to its maximum advantage, with frequent references to their failure in their first year of office. They pledged to consult the public a great deal in the process of health care reform. National criticised Labour for secrecy (National Archives, 1976c) and stressed the role of the general public in particular as important decision-makers.

National glossed over its previous failure when it tried to make significant changes in the health portfolio in the late 1960s and instead gained political capital from pointing out that it had previously created a Royal Commission to examine health care (National Archives, 1976c). The new reform effort officially began in May 1976, when it established the Special Advisory Committee on Health Services Organisation (SACHSO) to examine the organisation and coordination of health services. Following its election victory in 1975, National did not completely disband the groups working on issues relating to the White Paper, but asked them to complete their reports. Building on Labour's efforts, the SACHSO terms of reference reflected the emergent notion of health services as operating within a framework of preventive health care (Department of Health, 1982).

SACHSO was a product of both the White Paper failure and the electoral incentives that National faced. National, on the whole, was less ambitious than Labour in what it sought for the health sector. Unlike many Labour MPs, members of the National Government gave support to consumer choice and private sector medicine, although they wanted assurances people would not be disadvantaged through limited access to care or access only to second-class service (National Archives, 1976b). However, the government was careful to balance support for private medicine with reassurances that the public health system would remain. Perhaps National's stronger rural roots encouraged it to be more concerned about the localised nature of health care. National also learned from Labour's failure. The National Government framed the terms of reference for SACHSO delicately. The Committee was instructed to take communities of interest, traditional ties and geographical factors into consideration, while also considering the boundaries and responsibilities of hospital boards. The Minister of Health pledged to 'work through hospital boards' (Hansard, 1977). The government wanted to stress citizen participation in reform and promised community action centres to provide a 'grass roots level of communication between individuals and health services' (National Archives, 1983c).

Reform was deliberately consultative and incremental; it was also slow paced. National's health care reform was organised around committees on different health care topics. SACHSO spent the years between 1976 and 1978 deliberating on the best course of action before it put forward the first plan for health care reform. The government published a framework for discussion in 1977. SACHSO proposed replacing hospital boards with health boards that would be responsible for a wide range of services. Boards would be funded under global budgets and would replace district offices of the Department of Health. SACHSO proposed allowing the private and voluntary sectors a greater role in planning health services. A key part of the plan was diversity among localities and localised planning and involvement by citizens. Health care would be organised around particular kinds of health care services in different areas, such as paediatrics, geriatrics and mental health (Brookes, 1977). Between 1978 and 1982, the government tested its recommendations in pilot schemes in Northland and Wellington. The government claimed that policy-makers would look very closely at the outcomes of these pilot programmes.

In the 1970s, the National Government established multiple advisory boards in health care to advise the minister. By the early 1980s, ninety boards advised the Minister of Health (National Archives, 1982–84). The government had presumably learned from the White Paper that a successful reform plan could not ignore the political costs of appearing to impose plans on interest groups or local interests (Department of Health, 1982, p.6). Most importantly, the government adopted a sympathetic attitude towards the existing elected hospital board structures. SACHSO recommended that the initiative for health-care planning needed to come from 'those involved at the periphery, not a take-over, which vests the initiative in politicians or administrators at the centre' (Department of Health, 1982, p.6).

However, by the late 1970s options for health care reform were constrained by finance. Real public expenditure on health per person declined during the '70s. In 1970, public expenditure was NZ$1899 per person (in 1995 dollars), but by 1980 it was $1816 per person – a decline of -4.37 per cent, or just under half a per cent per year on average (OECD, 1999). Restraints on government spending were accepted by the Cabinet and introduced in the late 1970s. Financial ceilings were imposed (Hon. George F. Gair, 1980) and budget cuts, reductions in doctor and nurse training intakes, and rearrangements in the location of nurse training were made. Restraints were introduced in 1979 on growth of hospital budgets. Cabinet decided in December 1979 that government expenditure had to be considered within the context of the balance of payments deficit and goals of economic growth (National Archives, 1979).

Despite the financial constraints, the government was quietly hoping for major structural changes. By 1982, the Department of Health had established pilot programmes and completed a significant amount of groundwork in preparing the hospital sector for reform. It had also established an internal public relations committee (National Archives, 1980–82). In 1982, the Department of Health also suggested that SACHSO had entered a more 'political' phase that involved gaining the support of Cabinet and Caucus (National Archives, 1983c). Public acceptance of the proposals was also clearly on the minds of departmental advisers. The Department suggested that committees involved should assist in creating 'bottom-up' reform.

The release of National's reform plan

In late 1982, Minister of Health Aussie Malcolm released a fresh reform plan based on the SACHSO deliberations and pilot schemes (Department of Health, 1982). Prior to the release of the plan, he suggested that there was considerable support for health services reorganisation and the creation of Area Health Boards (AHBs), but that the reforms needed to be presented as a package. Although some suggest that the moves made by National essentially validated the White Paper, ministers were careful to avoid explicit mention of it (Martin, 1991, p.279). The Minister emphasised the need for extensive consultation and consensus seeking. Hospital boards were somewhat cautious because of their concerns regarding autonomy and their perception that there was little to be gained. The Department of Health reforms would have to be actively promoted (National Archives, 1983b). The Minister noted that unlike previous reorganisations, this one would not be imposed. Instead, it would proceed 'by the free will of hospital boards supported by the community' (National Archives, 1982a).

The reform plan proposed establishing AHBs comprised of constituent districts matching population to representation and with a mix of elected and appointed officials. There was no overt reference to amalgamation of boards, but Health Department officials hoped that AHBs would lead to the demise of at least the smallest boards. The government argued that the new boards should have a substantial majority of elected over appointed members. Area Health Boards were to be responsible for promoting the health of citizens within each community, including being responsible for planning health services in each area, involving communities in health services, and liaising with all organisations concerned with the promotion and maintenance of health. Boards would also be responsible for investigating and assessing the health needs of the community. The government suggested that transitions from hospital boards to AHBs could only be planned with the parties directly involved in the particular regional area. The 1982 reform plan proposed a Health Service Personnel Commission to act as the national personnel authority for staff employed in the health sector. The Commission would have the power to determine uniform and consistent personnel policies and, critically, to negotiate salary scales and conditions of employment. Government had to be sensitive to personnel issues because unions continued to be vocal throughout this period.

Many organisations submitted their responses to reform proposals in 1983. Groups as diverse as the Consumers' Union, the Employers' Federation, and a range of professional and hospital board associations presented submissions. There was more support for this plan than for the White Paper. Hospital boards were reluctant to see fundamental changes made, but not as vociferous as they had been in 1975. The Hospital Boards' Association supported the proposals in principle, but individual boards did not support change (National Archives, 1982b). Not all hospital boards made submissions. Six hospital boards were in favour of the proposed reorganisation. Three were against and five were uncommitted (National Archives, 1983a).

The Minister of Health, in co-operation with the Department of Health, had finally achieved some support for a change to the organisation and governance of AHBs. In 1983, legislation was introduced to enable hospital boards to change their status to AHBs. The Area Health Boards Act laid the foundation for further reform in the late 1980s (Martin, 1991, p.279). The 1983 legislation was a triumph in proposing larger boundaries for health administration, but the nature of the legislation was also largely at the discretion of hospital boards – they were not compelled to change their organisational status. The Act provided for the merger of hospital boards and district offices of the Department of Health to form AHBs, but only if local elected boards sought a merger. The legislation prescribed fundamental mandates for boards to be responsible for public health functions, co-ordination of all health services within an area, and established procedures for planning services at the local level. Finally, the legislation allowed for the appointment of board members if the elected members and the minister agreed (Martin, 1991, p.279). Boards did not exactly rush to be AHBs. Only two hospital boards had changed to AHB status by the end of 1985. The next chapter discusses the next stage in the slow process of developing regionally based health organisation through the 1980s.

Conclusion

Stronger partisan differences on health policy were evident after 1970. The Labour and National parties approached health care reform very differently. Whereas Labour entered office with ambitious plans, National's strategy in the late 1970s and early 1980s was to attempt incremental reform of the hospital sector only. National was not opposed to a public-private mix in health care and it avoided the pressing problem of how to pay and organise for primary health care. Labour, by contrast, saw the failure of the 1930s as the enduring problem of health care and continued to try to redress the difficulties of the past. National seemed unwilling to engage in the creation of a unified national health service. National's strategy was also less controversial than Labour's because it left primary care doctors, private insurers and voluntary organisations alone, and hence reduced significantly political tensions with the health sector. Labour's ill-fated 1974 reform plan had shown what could happen if governments proposed massive sector-wide reorganisation. Almost all groups had mobilised together to oppose change. In the 1970s, hospital boards had been helped by an expanding number of professional organisations, insurance companies, consumer groups and citizen organisations.

Local institutions also stalled the White Paper and SACHSO. The Labour Government's agenda of regionalisation of health care in New Zealand was challenged by the periphery. Local hospital boards continued to mobilise against changes in the hospital sector, and governments after 1975 learned to be wary of the power of the hospital boards. National learned from Labour's experience that it would need to work much harder to gain support from hospital boards and communities if they wanted to make structural changes to the national health service. The reform plan SACHSO released in 1982 was extremely cautious. Legislative change occurred, but the cost was time and compromise: legislation was not enacted until 1983 and it did not compel hospital boards to form AHBs. As the next chapter shows, it took Labour another six years to force the formation of AHBs.

CHAPTER **FIVE**

Inching towards marketisation, 1984 to 1990

THIS CHAPTER explores Labour's return to power in 1984 and its proposals for health care reform in 1987–88. Business leaders such as Alan Gibbs envisioned a more efficient health service modelled on the reformed railways and postal service. Yet, as in previous decades, these proposals met with local opposition. The chapter discusses why proposals for private-sector involvement in health care were ultimately jettisoned and why instead the 1989 Area Health Boards Act was passed, confirming the place of mixed elected/appointed boards.

Labour's election in July 1984 began a process of fundamental economic and policy reforms implemented over the next six years of their reign (James, 1992; Roberts, 1987). Hospital reform was part of their agenda. Two items in this agenda are examined in this chapter: the 1986 Health Benefits Review and the 1988 Taskforce on Hospital and Related Services (also known as the Gibbs Taskforce). These reform episodes promised to reform hospital and primary care arrangements and continued along the trajectory of previous reform efforts to address the geographical distribution of health care and the financial obstacles faced by primary care patients. The Health Benefits Review proposed many options, including competition between proposed health maintenance organisations and a system of government contracting with providers. The Gibbs Taskforce developed these models further and drew on lessons from economic reforms in the 1980s. Both reform efforts advanced the agenda for regional health services, but under the threat of much more radical proposals. As a result, Labour passed legislation that required hospital boards to merge into fourteen Area Health Boards (AHBs) in 1989.

Why did more market-oriented reforms emerge in the 1980s? As in other periods, health policy was influenced by changing ideas about government and economic conditions. Economic reforms were motivated by a sense of structural and economic crisis in New Zealand following the Muldoon era, and political support for new economic policies (Franklin, 1985). Voter support (Ellis, 1998; Nagel, 1998) for economic liberalisation was also stimulated by shifts in the traditional sources of support for the two major parties, and a coalition of support for reform (James, 1986; James, 1992). Voters became more likely to change allegiances in the late 1970s and early 1980s (Gold, 1986). New Zealand is widely perceived to have pursued economic liberalisation more extensively than most other countries (Boston, 1989; Easton and Gerritsen, 1996; Evans et al., 1996; Goldfinch, 2000; Kelsey, 1996; Roberts, 1987).

In other time periods, these larger forces affected the choices made and framed the general orientation of policy. In the 1980s, the links between economic policy, state sector reforms and health policies were forged anew. The apparent success of economic liberalisation in the 1980s made the government ambitious to apply the same theoretical framework for policy design in all areas of policy, even those that seemed to have long-standing problems and served quite different purposes, such as the hospital sector. There is robust evidence from archival documents (referenced in this chapter) that the same approach influenced the political understanding and policy options available. Frequently, Cabinet ministers referred to reform successes in other areas of the state sector as a justification for similar reforms in health. Just as the railways and postal services had been made more efficient, so could health services be commercialised for greater efficiency. Very different policy problems were considered identical and therefore thought to have similar solutions. The new sector-wide approach was inspired by a common set of understandings amongst officials in the leading departments (most notably Treasury), that liberalisation of the economy and state sector required attending to government rather than market failures (Boston, 1991).

This linkage can be seen in the players involved. A wider array of Cabinet ministers and officials with experience in economic liberalisation, rather than health only, were drawn into health care reform in the 1980s. As this chapter shows, this period differed because, for the first time in many years, the Department of Health was not developing a blueprint: Treasury took a significant role in the Gibbs Taskforce. The Department of Health was no longer the sole instigator or progenitor of ideas about how to reform health care.

Health Benefits Review 1986

Labour's paradigm for reform in the 1980s was one of radical change, and health care was no exception. Prime Minister David Lange said that the New Zealand health care system was 'locked into the most extraordinary patterns of the 1930s and require[d] a totally new approach' (National Archives, 1985a). Health care reform had allies in different factions of Cabinet, for different reasons. Ministers such as Finance Minister Roger Douglas were acutely sensitive to the power of special interests. Douglas argued there should be greater choice in health care, since doctors had not 'been given a God-given decree to solely administer to the sick' (Douglas, 1980). Both the left-wing and the right supported greater attention to public health and lifestyle causes of disease, perhaps for different reasons, but this provided a coalition of sorts. Health Minister Michael Bassett (between 1984 and 1987) was in favour of more competition in health care but disagreed with Douglas about how this was to be achieved (National Archives, 1981–86, National Archives, 1986b). He also stressed the need for more consumer-driven health care services (National Archives, 1987a).

In the early 1970s, the Department of Health had been instrumental in pursuing health care reform. The Department's main agenda in the 1980s was developing stronger public health policies. In the 1980s, Treasury took a leading role in health care reform, as it did in many policy areas. During that period, Treasury was able to 'set the broad philosophical and conceptual framework' for public policy debates in New Zealand (Boston, 1989, p.76). Treasury was an agency marked by its capacity to 'adopt a particular theoretical stance and then apply this as consistently as possible to the issues of the day' (Boston, 1989, p.76). (In New Zealand, as in Britain, the Treasury has the responsibility for both reviewing government expenditure and advising on economic policy.)

Treasury's analysis of the health care system between 1984 and 1985 appears to have been one factor that stimulated the formation of the Health Benefits Review in late 1985, but it was also the start of the greater agency focus on this policy area that was evident in the 1980s. Treasury stressed the need for greater efficiency in the sector and called for government to reconsider its rationale for state involvement in the sector (National Archives, 1987h). Treasury raised the question of whether health care goods were considered private, merit, public or luxury goods. (National Archives, 1987b). Treasury officials also wanted health services to be more responsive to citizens (National Archives, 1985b). In doing so it had taken up the mantle of the leftist critics of the 1970s, but for completely different reasons; the market system should be relied on for signals in terms of accountability of providers, and welfare benefits should be directed at individuals rather than providers (National Archives, p.195). The agency believed widespread reform would be necessary, from pharmaceutical benefits to fundamental changes in management structures and funding (National Archives, 1986c).

Once the decision was made to examine the health care sector, agencies debated the scope and terms of the inquiry. Agencies approached the task of health reform somewhat differently. Treasury used the framework of equity and efficiency in analysing health benefits. The Health Department proposed a term of reference for reform that mimicked the 1972 investigation into Social Security Benefits, and failed to address the framework increasingly being used by Treasury (National Archives, 1985c). By this stage, the Department of Health and the Board of Health had noticed that Treasury was interested in reforming the health arena and feared Treasury would make decisions without their contribution (National Archives, 1986a).

The final terms of reference included a review of health benefits in relation to goals of social and economic equity and efficiency, perhaps reflecting a compromise between the two agencies. To reduce the influence of interest groups (National Archives, 1985c), the government consciously avoided appointing direct interest group representatives to the Health Benefits Review. Instead, the government appointed a medical sociologist, an economist, and a general practitioner.

The review of health benefits presented a radical break from the past in terms of the analysis of the health care system and its approach to health care. Rather than providing a denunciation of the past followed by the presentation of the one and only best way forward, the analysis aimed to inform a broad public debate about health sector reform.[1] Overseas models influenced the reform options to a greater degree than in the past. The review team examined a large amount of literature on overseas health care, including literature on the Australian Medicare scheme, looked at the emerging health maintenance organisations in the United States, and consulted experts from around the world (National Archives, 1985–86). Although the Treasury was involved early-on, the agency did not get closely involved in the work of the Health Benefits Review on a day-to-day basis once it was established.

In keeping with all other efforts of reform that pointed to the previous failures to enact change, the Health Benefits Review report stressed the historical continuities in health policy. However, review members also argued for a new approach by analysing the health sector in new terms, involving the extent of state involvement in the health sector. A critical choice was whether to target providers or users (a supply versus demand approach to health care). The Health Benefits Review members chose to focus on providers, although they did suggest some means-testing in their recommendations for reform (National Archives, 1987q).

The Health Benefits Review concluded that there were five options for state involvement in health care. The options proposed included: options for competitive managed care; for minor changes to hospitals; changes to primary care benefits; a minimal safety-net role for government in health care; or for the state as a dominant funding source and provider. Option 4 was the preferred model, which incorporated state funding with provision shared between the government and private providers. Within Option 4 there were two subcategories. Option 4a advocated capitated payments for primary care. Option 4b allowed delegation of responsibility for health care to Area Health Boards.

The concept of 'Area Health Boards' that was included in Option 4 provided the government with maximum flexibility for future policy development. The proposals could be interpreted in different ways (National Archives, 1987–88c). Option 4 could seem like an interim step to less state involvement, but it could also be seen as an extension of public control over a wider sphere of health care (National Archives, 1987–88c).

Reaction to the Health Benefits Review

The Health Benefits Review won support by combining a concern for better public health outcomes with a desire for efficiency, a strategy that won it support from the public health community and from those arguing for more scrutiny of public expenditure. The review also emphasised the need for consumer choice beyond mainstream 'Western' medicine and thus appealed to groups who felt marginalised in the health care system. This was a winning political strategy. The careful use of evidence in the report and deliberative style won favour among academics.

Cabinet gave the appearance of being committed to change. Prior to the 1987 election, the Minister of Health stated he wanted a primary care health policy immediately following the election (National Archives, 1987e). A new Minister of Health, David Caygill, took over from Michael Bassett in 1987. Once in office, Caygill indicated that he supported a variation of Option 4b (National Archives, 1988m). However, within Cabinet, there were differences in opinion about the report. Treasury and the Minister of Finance opposed the findings of the report and objected to the fact that it had failed to deal with hospitals.

Submissions from the public suggested support for Option 4, especially 4b, which was a natural progression of the continuing efforts in New Zealand to create a greater regional orientation in health care. However, reform authors had wisely been opaque regarding the implications of AHBs contracting for primary care, and therefore doctors were less critical than in previous reform efforts. Nurse groups joined in, both asking for more benefits and stressing equality of access as a core value. The New Zealand Nurses' Association (NZNA) advocated a salaried medical service and a widening of eligibility to other health professionals, and the Chief Nurses of New Zealand supported Option 4b (National Archives, 1987c).

Many groups saw reform as the best way for them to gain government subsidies. Groups speaking on behalf of patients and those with specific health conditions, and health providers ranging from providers of long-term care to midwives made a case for broadening subsidies beyond doctors (National Archives, 1986d). Many organisations lobbied for government support, particularly those providing natural therapies. Private insurers also argued for greater choice in health care and private hospital providers argued against removal of government subsidies for private hospital care. Letters from members of the public suggest that most voters who were motivated to write to the Minister of Health supported 4 or 4b (National Archives, 1987c). Opinion polls suggested that the public was not extraordinarily worried about the health system. Citizens were unhappy with waiting lists but were not actively pressuring government for reform. Two-thirds of the respondents of one survey regarded the standard of care provided by public hospitals as very good or excellent (National Research Bureau, 1986).

Policy effects of the Health Benefits Review

Surprisingly, the level of consensus on the need for health care reform and relatively constructive debates about various options among interest groups, academics and the government did not materialise into health care reform. The Health Benefits Review recommendations did not result in a great policy transformation. As in previous times, Labour's hesitancy was a reflection of longstanding nervousness about the problems of rationalising hospitals, which more or less divided politicians along ideological lines.

The main area of contention within Cabinet appears to have been rationalisation of providers at the local level (National Archives, 1988m). Labour experienced significant conflict between members of Cabinet who supported the liberalisation programme and the ministers who wanted social policy generosity to balance the negative effects of structural adjustment (New Zealand Medical Journal, 1988). Health Minister David Caygill won the support of market reformers by promising to institute structural change in the hospital system, but this was not achieved in the way ministers such as Roger Douglas probably would have liked. Douglas argued that rationalisation was necessary because the objectives of board members differed from those of the government (National Archives, 1988m) and did not need to consider the needs of the health sector nationally.

The review increased health benefits and co-payments in some areas of primary care, but its direct effects on hospitals were less important. Its main effect was to change the framing of the health care debate by raising the possibility of creating competitive health maintenance plans. The taskforce further reinforced the idea of regionally based organisations and its framework for analysing the health care system reverberated throughout the late 1980s and 1990s (Scott, 1989). The Health Benefits Review also brought equity and efficiency explicitly into consideration as two fundamental policy goals and raised questions regarding the expenditure of public funds on health care, the lack of quality or efficiency indicators, and the bias towards institutional care over community or primary care. The authors suggested that both general practitioners and public hospitals should be more accountable to the public and government (Scott et al., 1989).

As a result of the Health Benefits Review, the Labour Government developed better accountability frameworks for hospitals and a stronger role for public health. The Government established New Zealand Health Goals in 1989, which included a reduction in smoking, improved nutrition, reduction in alcohol consumption, and reduction in mortality and morbidity resulting from motor vehicle accidents. Support for public health goals by the Government was a strategic way of ensuring better hospital board compliance under the guise of improved health outcomes. Those boards who were against better health outcomes risked looking too attached to the curative model.

The Taskforce on Hospital and Related Services, 1987

The Health Benefits Review had not focused on hospitals. The Taskforce on Hospital and Related Services was established in early 1987, close to the completion of the Health Benefits Review. The official rationale was that an additional inquiry into hospitals was needed. Another possible explanation is that some Cabinet members were dissatisfied with the failure of the Health Benefits Review to address the hospital system.

The Taskforce on Hospital and Related Services was established to investigate the management structures within hospitals and government funding to hospitals. The Taskforce started as a discussion between Alan Gibbs, who would later be the leader of the taskforce, and Finance Minister Roger Douglas. Gibbs boasted that he could save 33 per cent of the health budget. Douglas asked him to undertake the review (Mannion, 1987). Its recommendations were influenced by the reform of public trading companies, business practices, and ideas about commercial efficiency. Finance Minister Roger Douglas worked more closely with the Taskforce than with the Health Benefits Review. He was mindful of provider capture in health care (Douglas, 1980; National Archives, 1987v) and he strongly supported consumer choice. He argued that many health professionals supported reform but were cynical after multiple reviews over forty years had made little progress (National Archives, c1987).

Treasury was working on its own review of hospitals before the Taskforce was established (National Archives, 1988g), and the documentary evidence suggests Treasury may have excluded officials from the Department of Health from discussions (National Archives, 1986c) and revised policy papers because of professional sensitivities before circulating them to other agencies (National Archives, 1986c). Treasury made key decisions regarding the terms of reference and direction early on in the reform process (National Archives, 1987k). Its officials envisaged the review as being similar to the United Kingdom's 'Griffith' proposals to reform the National Health Service (National Archives, 1987j). Treasury performed most of the analyses for the Taskforce under instruction from its members (National Archives, 1987p).

The Taskforce was surrounded by controversy (Scott, 1989) and its deliberations were frequently leaked to the media, which only served to increase debate about its work. Groups on the left were particularly critical that businessman Alan Gibbs was chosen to lead it. Many interest groups thought this was a signal that the Labour Government would privatise health care, and the Labour Party lobbied for removing Alan Gibbs (National Archives, 1987e). One union described Gibbs as a 'Trojan horse looking to transfer health care into the vultures of the private sector' (National Archives, 1987z). Undeterred, Roger Douglas argued that union opposition was evidence that greater efficiency was necessary in the health services (National Archives, 1987e). The Department of Health proposed additional Taskforce members. Dame Dorothy Fraser and Professor John Scott were added, who brought hospital board and clinical experience, respectively, to the deliberations. Both were known for their sympathy and support for the public health system (Scott, 1989).

Politicians and Treasury officials verbally instructed Taskforce members on their preferred conclusions. They did not want written distribution of the materials and 'oral briefing of the consultants would be more important in determining the content of the report' (National Archives, 1987i). Treasury's view was that a three-month timetable, or a 'short, sharp approach', as they described it, would facilitate rapid change (National Archives, 1987j). Ministers were determined that, this time, *reform would happen*. Roger Douglas and Health Minister Michael Bassett had said they did not want the review to simply add to the existing pile of paper (National Archives, 1987v). They warned Taskforce members that 'health or health care reform has always been a difficult and painful process. Health is a subject which attracts much public and political attention, rendering reform very much a public debate' (National Archives, 1988d). But Taskforce members had been told their task was a 'no holds barred' review (National Archives, 1987b).

Deliberations of the Taskforce

Not unlike the Health Benefits Review, the Taskforce members began the deliberations with a discussion of the role of the state. However, the discussion at this review had a more ideological tint. Alan Gibbs argued that collectivism had been proved around the world as being insensitive or inefficient compared with the market, and the question was whether society had a corporate responsibility for all its members. The public expected a 'cradle to the grave' welfare state and free hospital facilities in an emergency. Consumers were attached to government intervention in health care. According to some Taskforce members, who discussed their observations of what consumers had told them, consumers wanted access to free hospitals and locally available services, 'like the post office: part of the fabric of the community' (National Archives, 1987), and although consumers did not voice their demands, they wanted better management, organisational change, and responsive institutions. Officials stressed that the Taskforce should not offend voters by suggesting that services could be cut, again showing the political sensitivities around cutting services or closing hospitals:

> This must not be seen as a cost-cutting issue, but as a re-allocation of resources, otherwise it will be opposed ... Hospitals are part of the fabric of what New Zealanders regard as facilities that comprise a community. Threats of closure are met with considerable community concern (National Archives, 1987).

History showed that reform had indeed been difficult. Taskforce officials and members referred to earlier inquiries, such as the White Paper of 1975, and analysed difficulties in the health sector in the post-war period. Financial accountability in hospitals was mainly concerned with over- or under-allocation (National Archives, 1987b), and laws prescribing the activities of hospital boards placed disproportionate emphasis on national approval. Treasury noted that confused relationships existed between the boards and the Department of Health. The Department of Health gave guidelines for health services to hospitals, but offered no incentives for changing practices (National Archives, 1986c). Hospital boards had originally been responsible only for hospital care, one report noted, but over time expectations developed for increased spending on preventive, community and primary services (National Archives, 1987u). Elected boards were criticised for their parochial outlook and lack of management skills. The existence of New Zealand's smallest hospital boards (Table 4) showed the persistence of the board structures over time, taskforce members argued.

Taskforce staff stressed the parochial interests of boards and, in particular, their interest in preserving local facilities. They noted that board facilities were attractive issues for MPs to be associated with, and that ministers were sensitive to these needs (National Archives, 1987u). Thus:

Table 4. Smaller hospital boards, 1987

Board name	Population
Maniototo	2,800
Waiapu	4,850
Vincent	11,900
Taumarunui	12,900
Central Hawkes Bay	13,050
Dannevirke	13,100
South Otago	16,600
Waitaki	21,500
Ashburton	24,800

Source: National Archives (National Archives, 1987u)

Sensible regional arrangements can only be developed by reducing the influence of such boards, or a more drastic approach, the elimination of many small or medium boards and the development of a few large regional bodies with comprehensive responsibilities (National Archives, 1987u).

The Taskforce quickly developed two models for the health system that informed their subsequent analysis: (1) central government funding, and (2) a consumer-funding model (National Archives, 1987r). By June 1987, they had concluded that separation of provision from funding was essential and, internally, the consumer model remained a serious option. However, ministers were advised to be coy in dealings with the media and were told to keep their options open (National Archives, 1987d). The development of two models served to show some fault-lines within the Taskforce (National Archives, 1987p). Alan Gibbs supported an insurance model, with means-tested assistance provided through the Department of Social Welfare. Meanwhile, Taskforce member John Scott was a supporter of Area Health Boards but also saw the difficulty of local communities overriding central government. He considered the possibility of competing insurance organisations (state and market) for New Zealand. Dorothy Fraser suggested funding the health care system through a separate tax would indicate to consumers how much they were paying for health care (National Archives, 1987p).

Taskforce options for the health care system were largely based on the policy analysis performed by seconded officials, overseas economists and private sector consultants. But some of the experts who reviewed the options said the work was flawed. For example, policy analysts thought people would travel to find the best care and insurers would fund choice: 'we would expect to see much greater flows across existing board boundaries as people went to the specialist who best met their particular requirements ... the insurance company would have an incentive' to find the most appropriate provider for those patients (National Archives, 1988f). The Taskforce also used an Arthur Andersen and Company report, endorsed by the Director General of Health (National Archives, 1988e), which suggested that cost savings of up to 30 per cent would result from health care reform. The Health Minister David Caygill later admitted in Parliament in June 1988 that the savings were based on 'very poor data'. The study was widely considered to be flawed; it failed to control for patient differences between hospitals and confused average and marginal costs (National Archives, 1987–88a; National Archives, 1988b; National Archives, 1988l).

Overseas academics recommended that New Zealand take a cautious approach to health care reform. Harold Luft, an economist and expert on health maintenance organisations, agreed that existing local hospitals were too small to be efficient (National Archives, 1987o). However, he was pessimistic about the opportunities for competition in New Zealand's small market because of the potential for collusion among tertiary care providers. He questioned whether competing plans would be set up in other parts of the country, or if health maintenance organisations would be able to offer tertiary care to residents of other areas. Luft suggested that competition could appropriate eventually but in the short term regionally based health maintenance organisations would be advisable (National Archives, 1987o). Luft also cautioned that insurers could avoid enrolling those people who required extensive treatment or could use marketing to attract good risks (National Archives, 1987o).

Anthony Culyer, an economist from the University of York, was even more critical of the policy analysis. Some pages of the report 'amazed and disturbed', said Culyer. 'They are full of false assertions and half truths' (National Archives, 1987s). Culyer recommended slower changes and said that New Zealand's performance was more favourable on most available indicators of input and output than the Taskforce had suggested. He also recommended against the development of prepaid health maintenance organisations. Adverse selection would make equity objectives difficult to meet (National Archives, 1987s), echoing comments made by Luft. A plan to introduce competition would require regulation to prevent adverse selection, thus destroying the benefits of competition. Finally, Culyer argued that the competitive insurance model would not solve problems of lack of efficiency in the delivery sectors (National Archives, 1987s).

Luft and Culyer were more sceptical than Treasury officials regarding the benefits of competition and the potential for efficiency. Treasury believed that choice would be desirable for consumers, who could choose the services they wanted nearby: 'They may be prepared to travel some distance, say to Auckland, as at present, or may not want some types of service at all' (National Archives, 1988f). However, experts' concerns reflected existing economic theories of insurance markets (Rothschild and Stiglitz, 1976) that were later elaborated in the 1990s (Newhouse, 1994), since plans will develop ways to attract good risks either through segmentation, benefit selection, co-payment levels, or marketing (Newhouse, 1996). Hospitals could bid services away from each other, which might result in declining levels of services that the system was supposed to provide.

Although some of this scholarship was not yet published, not all of the expert advice received by the Taskforce was adopted, although the Taskforce did reject the fully consumer-driven model. By around October 1987, the Taskforce had developed a model where a central health commission would transfer funds to Area Health Boards. These boards would provide a full range of services with the exception of primary care. People could opt out and receive coverage from approved private insurers and would receive a tax rebate or grant. Boards would not provide treatment services but would contract with providers. This policy was based on assumptions such as adequate risk adjustment and competitive neutrality between state and insurers (National Archives, 1987w), assumptions that appeared to pay lip service to the advice they received from Culyer and Luft. Hospitals and other providers would operate on a commercial basis (National Archives, 1987t). Taskforce members considered that separating funding and provision would reduce or end principal-agent problems in health care.

Resolving the tensions between commercial and democratic principles was difficult. Health Minister David Caygill supported elected, not appointed, officials (1987a) and Taskforce members held slightly different views about the best way to restructure boards (National Archives, 1987f), especially Fraser and Gibbs. Dame Fraser thought boards should be restructured with some appointed and some elected members because voters liked to feel that they had influence on governing the health services (National Archives, 1987f; National Archives, 1987m). John Scott favoured regions and larger boards, because elected hospital boards had a personal stake in general in fighting for their own survival and had a very limited overview of the changes that were necessary nationally. He opposed vouchers, given the 'emotional and prejudiced attitudes to vouchers', and said he favoured Options 3 and 4 set out in the Health Benefits Review (National Archives, 1987m).

Overall, Taskforce members were mostly pessimistic that changes could be made in the short term; Scott and Gibbs took a more long-term view. Scott suggested that the Taskforce would probably be able to influence the political climate so that politicians would feel less constrained in making necessary changes. Gibbs thought privatisation would be possible over twenty years: '... the country has not reached the stage where it is prepared to see anyone go without health care. It may be possible in 20 years time' (National Archives, 1987f). He thought in the future that Area Health Boards would provide 'the safety net' (National Archives, 1988o). 'The long-term goal would be a more market-oriented approach', in a minimum of five years (National Archives, 1987l). Scott considered change would occur in decades (National Archives, 1987q) and he argued that revolution was not desirable.

Fraser and Scott tried to learn about community preferences and visited towns throughout the country. According to Fraser and Scott, people in small communities said they believed they had a right to health care services nearby, and were fearful that corporatisation of hospitals would lead to privatisation; they held out for continued local autonomy (National Archives, 1987g). Rural groups rallied against centralisation of health care services. Communities were resistant to appointed boards, and defended the use of elections for board members. Citizens said they liked to feel they were contributing to decision-making.

This feedback may have led the Taskforce to consider issuing shares in hospital chains to the public. This was seen as a more politically acceptable way to avoid opposition from members of the public to 'their' hospital being taken over. Privatisation was presented as the best option for efficiency reasons, but the unpopularity of privatisation was noted, suggesting a corporatisation trial might be appropriate (National Archives, 1987y). Scott expressed reservations about the competition model working in some areas of the country and suggested that cultural and social features of New Zealand would lead to resistance to market-oriented changes. He suggested making the present system more efficient as a first step in the proposed sequence which, he felt, would make it unnecessary to develop more commercialised models later (National Archives, 1987l).

Meanwhile, speculation was growing in the press, frequently based on leaked Taskforce documents. The social democratic wing of the Parliamentary Labour Party was dissatisfied and complained that the Labour Government's caucus committee was stacked to favour market solutions for health care (Clark, 1987a). Most interest groups and individual submissions to the Taskforce showed support for a public hospital system (National Archives, 1987b). Very few groups were in favour of increasing means-testing or introducing vouchers. However, support was growing for hospital reform. The overwhelming majority – apart from professionals – wanted to reform the management system of hospitals, that was dominated by professionals. Doctors favoured management by doctors and hospital managers favoured the development of a new managerial class (New Zealand Medical Association, 1987–88).

On 6 November 1987, the Taskforce met and discussed a draft version of its report, in which two models were presented (National Archives, 1987n). The first was a government-owned or sponsored insurer of right, with regional boards funding or providing services not covered by the national insurance agency. The national insurer would compete with other funders in a neutral environment for various health services and would allow people to opt out. A second option proposed a system of regional health boards which would be responsible for the total health care in each area, and could operate as insurers or as health maintenance organisations in a competitively neutral environment. People would also be able to opt out of this arrangement.

A few weeks later, another meeting considered the final Taskforce report. Gibbs felt that the final report focused entirely on management and structural change and did not raise value judgements, and proposed the minimum change possible to existing institutions and structures (National Archives, 1988c). Treasury officials advised the Taskforce to carefully consider the wording of the report and to consider recommending a more radical approach, to give politicians 'room to manoeuvre'. In addition, they advised the authors to present extreme options that they had discarded, because readers would expect the Taskforce to recommend these as options. Treasury warned against executive summaries that would be 'the focus of uninformed comment and debate' in the media (National Archives, 1987–88b). Alan Gibbs suggested that the report should focus on the terms of reference and on hospitals, and that it should build on momentum for Area Health Board concepts (National Archives, 1988a).

Meanwhile, the Minister of Health David Caygill advised the Cabinet Social Equity Committee that he expected a negative reception for the report and considerable media interest (National Archives, 1988j). He discussed how the Taskforce's non-public style had irked pressure groups: 'The small information that has filtered out from the Taskforce's discussions has tended to confirm their worst fears' (National Archives, 1988j). In particular, employee groups had continued to have a negative view of the Taskforce, while hospital administrators and boards would be unlikely to welcome the report since any recommendations for improvements to the existing system would probably be interpreted as criticisms of the present management. Caygill said: 'At best, Hospital Boards are likely to be defensive' (National Archives, 1988j). Tellingly, he commented that, regardless of whether Cabinet was intending to implement the report, it would be important to encourage a positive attitude to change in the health sector (National Archives, 1988j). To prepare the public for the criticisms of the Taskforce, staff of the Minister of Finance worked to find local examples of hospital mismanagement to give to MPs and selected journalists. The office warned that local hospital boards would be defensive and would obfuscate and deny problems (National Archives, 1988h).

Policy papers produced through the summer of 1987 and 1988 continued to advocate a stronger role for price signals in the health system. In December 1987, one policy paper stressed the need for privatisation, given a desire for efficiency, while also acknowledging the opposition of community groups. Instead, officials suggested that two or three hospitals could be commercialised (National Archives, 1987y). In February 1988, the Taskforce was still intent on a considerably commercialised model of health care, but without entitlement transfer between the state and private insurers. Taskforce participants were still considering mentioning a system of targeted health benefits at a later stage. Under this future plan, insurance would be individually based and the insurance industry would be unregulated. Area Health Boards would be used for providing services to the needy and would act as the safety net (National Archives, 1988o).

Once released, the final Taskforce report was considerably different from these drafts. Both the language and the nature of the policy proposals themselves had been muted considerably. The report avoided explicit discussion of targeting, and was more opaque about the future direction of the health care system. The Taskforce report was named *Unshackling the Hospitals* (New Zealand Hospital & Related Services Taskforce, 1988). The report detailed the management deficiencies of hospitals and posed a split between funding and provision of health care to encourage efficiency. The authors acknowledged that their model was derived from the Health Benefits Review Option 4b, but the Taskforce rejected this option in the final report. The government wished to remain the dominant funder of health services. Therefore, the authors recommended that government should distribute funds to a national health commission. The commission would allocate funds to six regional health authorities and primary health care providers, monitor the performance of regional health authorities, and undertake research and evaluation on the health sector as a whole. Regional Health Authorities (RHAs) would be 'lean independent elected bodies with small operating budgets and tightly defined duties' and would be responsible for buying services for their areas. The report was coy about primary care and simply said that, at a later date, primary care could be reviewed and providers would be encouraged to co-operate with the regional health authorities.

Reaction to reform proposals and interest group submissions

The Gibbs Report, as it came to be known, started and ended its deliberations with considerable media attention. The reaction to the Gibbs Report by many interest groups was not favourable, despite the efforts to make the report less controversial before its release, and despite the effort made to consult some groups. The report was perceived as a first step in the privatisation of health care. Health Minister David Caygill distanced himself from the Taskforce and denied that the report had been 'toned down' at the direction of the Labour Government. He said that he had instructed the Taskforce that they should not feel constrained by his views or those of his colleagues, and he made arguments as to why health care was 'different' (National Archives, 1988n). Prime Minister David Lange was reported as saying that user pays was opposite to Labour policy (Clark, 1987b). Labour Party President Margaret Wilson had previously said that health care would not be sold like other commodities and that it was a basic human right. David Lange said previously that he had never doubted the role of the state as the primary funder of health care and stressed that 'you can't have people dying for lack of money' (1987b). He also said education and health could not be cut (National Archives, 1988k).

Hospital boards were now in a difficult situation. The Hospital Boards' Association had been given a firm message by the Minister of Health in May 1987 that maintenance of the status quo was not an option. He told board chairpeople that there were only three options for the health service: first, doing nothing, with boards risking being commercialised; second, developing a two-tier system; or third, acceptance in principle that there would be a reduction in the number of boards (National Archives, 1988i). The chair of the Hospital Boards' Association had said that they accepted that some hospitals would translate into Area Health Boards (AHBs) quite readily but argued that some other boards would need to have discussions (National Archives, 1988i). By October 1987, the Hospital Boards' Association was clearly concerned about its viability, given the scope of the Taskforce and was claiming that AHBs would be well placed to undertake responsibility for funding, obtaining and providing primary health care (National Archives, 1987x). However, despite these statements, the boards continued to be slow in transferring to AHB status. By the end of 1987, only four hospital boards out of twenty-nine had taken up the offer of transferring to an AHB structure.

Policy Effects of the Taskforce

Labour did not adopt the policies advocated by Gibbs but gained a great deal from the Taskforce report. The Government distanced itself from the report findings, while using the report as a threat to extract gains that had been planned for decades. Post-Gibbs, the Labour Government had a powerful ultimatum and considerable leverage over hospital boards and thus between 1986 and 1990 increased its control. The Minister of Health continued previous reform efforts in terms of advocating regionalisation and accountability. What had began as a potentially radical taskforce with libertarian leadership ultimately became a tool of the more left-leaning factions in the Labour Cabinet.

David Caygill introduced a plan called 'Health: A Prescription for Change' in 1988 to require boards to negotiate budgets and performance criteria with central government. Eventually, boards would assume responsibility for primary care planning and funding. The devolution of primary care was not, in fact, implemented (Martin, 1991). A new Minister of Health, Helen Clark, was appointed in 1989 and she continued to increase hospital board accountability for public health. She introduced the New Zealand Health Charter, which contained public health goals such as reducing smoking and improving nutrition. Clark also initiated a system of performance contracts to be signed by the Minister of Health and the chairperson of the AHBs (Martin, 1991). Between 1989 and 1990, contracts were signed between AHBs and the Minister that required boards to be responsible for health outcomes (Ashton, 1992). The 1983 Area Health Boards Act was amended to allow the Minister to appoint board members, a policy supported by numerous previous governments. However, this initiative was not taken until 1991.

The government was finally able to make stronger demands on hospital boards and engage in some rationalisation of administrative functions, justifying them as necessary for the improvement of health outcomes. Hospital boards were reorganised into fourteen AHBs under changes to local government legislation in 1989. Boards were encouraged to draw some lessons from the Gibbs report in improving information systems and management structures. Martin notes that the structure of accountability relationships remained an unusual mix of local accountability and central funding (Martin, 1991). The accountability of boards to local communities remained a problem of the emerging structure around 1989 and 1990 (Davies, 1989). These tensions continued to pose difficulties that precipitated the reforms of 1991 considered in the next chapter.

By 1989, Cabinet had made some preliminary moves to combine certain health care districts (National Archives, 1982–90) after Health Minister David Caygill introduced changes to procedures for funding allocations of AHBs. The Government introduced greater accountability requirements with the passage of the Area Health Boards Amendment Act (1989). Contracts with boards were introduced that were outcome-focused and public health-oriented rather than being provider contracts. User charges for medicines were increased, but Cabinet rejected the system of competitive funding.

Conclusion

Of the two reform episodes considered here, the Gibbs Taskforce is frequently considered to have been more influential because National later adopted some of the ideas in this report, and because some changes sequentially followed the Gibbs Report. In some ways, the Health Benefits Review was equally important during the term of the Labour Government as it encouraged a more aggressive policy towards regionalisation and accountability.

The 1980s saw central government lose its patience with the incremental strategies used in the past. Ultimately, however, boards were retained and embedded within the new structures that emerged through the decade, confirming their central role in the New Zealand health system. The government forced boards to become more accountable and forced the amalgamation of boards into Area Health Boards. Labour also created the *environment* for National to make much more fundamental changes to the structure of hospital boards in the 1990s. Labour's achievement was that, by foreshadowing significant change, it was able to obtain greater control over hospital boards and regionalisation. This was a winning strategy because both hospital boards and the public feared more fundamental reform. After the spectre of partial privatisation, the Labour Government's plans for health care in terms of regionalism seemed relatively benign. Labour foreshadowed privatisation through the Gibbs Taskforce and then was able to introduce considerably more moderate reforms under the guise of improving public health. Although the Area Health Board Act had been in place since 1983, only a handful of boards had converted by 1987 and they would not have changed their status voluntarily.

Economic reform influenced the environment for health reform in important ways. There were tactical advantages. Labour capitalised its resolve to override interest group pressure in other areas of the economy. Labour's success in other areas of policy reform made it appear tough and uncompromising. However, in other ways economic reform might have made health interest groups wary and ready to mobilise against change. Finally, the economic reforms of the 1980s were notable for their divisive impact within the Labour Party, causing leadership changes and tensions between Roger Douglas and David Lange, while the left-of-centre faction within Labour protected social policy and health. This protection was lost after 1990, when National was able to act with much more ideological unity in its efforts at reform, as discussed in the next chapter.

CHAPTER **SIX**

The end of elected boards

THE NATIONAL PARTY was elected into power in November 1990 and in 1991 the new government proposed a design for a new health sector based on competition between public and private providers, with regional purchasers. The reform outline also proposed the introduction of a managed competition system of competing health care plans. The *coup de grace* of the 1990s was to be the government's success in ending local representation on Area Health Boards (AHBs). Cabinet used the institutions of New Zealand's Westminster system to remove the most troublesome feature of the health care system, which had made hospital reform almost impossible during the twentieth century. However, the end of local representation also inspired an unexpected public reaction against the government's entire reform programme (Gauld, 2000; Laugesen, 2005, p.6).[1] The National Government had mixed success and many aspects of the reform process were hampered by controversy, including patient co-payments for public hospitals, the standard benefits package, vouchers for private insurance, and commercialised hospitals.

This chapter analyses three phases of the reform process: from the initial development and announcement of reform through to the implementation and revision of policy in 1996–97. During implementation, intense political pressure called on National to curtail reform. To mitigate this negative reaction, ministers used a range of strategies to shape the public

---

1. Some of the material in this chapter draws on Laugesen (2005).

debate on reform. The survival of policies is considered in the last part of the chapter, which suggests that even National's elimination of elected boards did not solve or reduce the political conflicts in the hospital sector.

Reform beginnings

National gave contradictory signals about its intention to reform health care during the 1990 election campaign, telling the press it would increase the role of the private sector and impose commercial discipline on public hospitals (1987). Its manifesto promised the continuation of AHBs with elected and appointed members (Ashton, 1992). Greater support of private hospitals was consistent with National's support of the private hospital industry since the 1950s, and introduced tax exemptions for private insurance in the 1960s. Since 1987, the party had been supportive of greater use of market incentives in health care. Between 1987 and 1990, National Party policy was moving towards a greater role in health care for the private sector. While in Opposition, Ruth Richardson, who became Finance Minister, proposed a welfare state with a minimal safety-net (National Archives, 1987), and an influential group in caucus was known to favour a residual approach to welfare provision (Boston et al., 1999).

National's platform on health care once it entered government continued along a trajectory of lesser state involvement. A taskforce was appointed in December 1990 to develop recommendations that would reduce the role of the state in health care, increase efficiency and choice in the health service, and increase responsiveness to consumers. Officials and ministers involved in directing the taskforce suggested: '… The eventual goal is a society in which the state is only required to offer support for a small proportion of the population and where most people accept responsibility for themselves and their families' (National Archives, c1991). Competition at all levels was the mechanism proposed to achieve this goal. A draft terms of reference stated that the assumed role of public health policy was to reduce the government's fiscal risk, rather than to improve health outcomes (Ministry of Health, 1991b).

Taskforce officials established a blueprint for reform in two months, by February 1991. They developed reform options in relative isolation from the Department of Health but worked closely with ministers. Ministers preferred to limit discussion to selected ministers and sympathetic officials. For example, initial reform papers in December 1990 were sent to Treasury but not the Director General of the Department of Health (Ministry of Health, 1990). National ministers wanted to announce reform in the July Budget of 1991 and implement change quickly (National Archives, 1991b).[2] Some officials had reservations about the timetable and wanted to warn ministers that a short deadline would constrain the work programme (National Archives, 1991c). The time available and the style of policy development probably reduced the number of alternatives explored and the depth of policy research undertaken.

The process invites comparisons with the Clinton plan of 1993 in the United States, in terms of time constraints and style of policy development, with most proposals being developed between January and May 1993 (Skocpol, 1996), and with relative exclusivity. In both countries, the secrecy surrounding health care reform appeared to alienate interest groups and the public. A recurring theme in the hundreds of submissions later made by professionals and the public to the New Zealand government was the need for wider, more comprehensive involvement in the development of policy proposals (Department of Prime Minister and Cabinet, 1992).

By May 1991, the taskforce had developed a proposal for the separation of financing health care and its provision: Regional Health Authorities (RHAs) would contract with providers of health services, including hospitals and private businesses.[3] Individuals could opt out of RHAs, allowing competition between insurers. Uniform user charges were proposed. Risk-adjusted social insurance would 'encourage people to live healthier lives because they would have a greater incentive to live well, avoid accidents, economise on their use of health services and save for the health costs of old age.' Social insurance would provide a 'signal [to each person for] how much health expenditure it thinks is appropriate', 'greater certainty of funding for the health sector, greater diversity of sources of funding and better incentives for self care, cost-effective care and saving for the health care costs of old age' (Ministry of Health, 1991c). Reduced government expenditure was expected through such insurance, and cost-shifting onto patients was expected to generate fiscal savings of $1 billion per year. The disadvantages of these proposals included a long and costly implementation process and potential for social insurance to be unpopular

2. The health taskforce's work plan was constrained by the timing of the July Budget.
3. The taskforce officials noted the similarities between reforms of state-owned enterprises and the health service, where state-owned businesses were reformed and expected to produce returns on assets.

with voters (Ministry of Health, 1991f).

The Office of the Prime Minister and Cabinet tried to estimate the advantages and disadvantages of reform. They thought reform would lead to clearer roles and objectives for funders and providers, incentives for providers and funders to be efficient and responsive to consumers, less dominance by hospital providers in securing resources, greater local control of hospitals, and reduced waiting times. The expected costs included staff reductions, reorganisation of resources within AHBs, revision of legislation and regulations, establishment of various new organisations, and monitoring arrangements. Costs were described as immediate implementation costs that would produce efficiency gains in the medium to longer term (Ministry of Health, 1991c, pp.6–7).

By June 1991, a proposal for reform gave extensive justification for ending local representation on AHBs. The officials considered that reform was necessary because AHBs had few incentives to manage their assets prudently; they could simply under-service patients when budgets were tight, rather than manage resources more efficiently. Conflicting accountabilities to both local electors and the Minister of Health meant that AHBs faced further difficulties. Ownership of AHBs also subjected the government to 'fiscal risk'. The taskforce considered the current board system unworkable because there was an 'inescapable conflict of interest that arises because elected board members have local accountability while their resources are derived from central government revenue' (Ministry of Health, 1991c). Furthermore, the taskforce concluded that elected boards had provided neither direction for management of hospital services nor effective representation of consumer concerns. Instead, it proposed that public hospital providers be established as autonomous businesses, with boards of directors appointed by the government. Consumers could opt out of the government insurance plan once RHBs were operational, allowing citizens to possibly use a voucher. Officials hoped that pre-paid insurance plans could be introduced in July 1993.

The National Government knew that there would be considerable opposition to the plan to reform AHBs. Advisers thought that it would 'require careful management of the transition from current arrangements to new structures, and clear communication ...' (Ministry of Health, 1991c, p.5) and that the Minister of Health should make changes swiftly, replacing board members with appointees as soon as reform was announced. There was a risk that board members would 'obstruct reform, and take action that would seriously compromise the Crown's ownership interest in boards' (Ministry of Health, 1991c). Advisers recommended legislation be introduced under urgency to 'permit appointment of Commissioners in these circumstances' (Ministry of Health, 1991c). Cabinet agreed to follow this advice.

The Minister of Finance, Ruth Richardson, promised that she would present a 'Mother of all Budgets' in July 1991, and hinted that it would provide the framework for all government policies, including social policy. On the night of the Budget reading in Parliament, the Minister of Health presented the health reform plan (Ministry of Health, 1991h). It was introduced as part of a social welfare package, 'Welfare that Works', and argued for significant change on the grounds that AHBs lacked clarity regarding which services hospital boards were required to provide (Ministry of Health, 1991h). It proposed the introduction of a standard benefits package, commercialisation of public providers, and four regional purchasers that would contract with providers. Private insurers could compete with government health care purchasers for government funding.

That same night, legislation was introduced under urgency rules to remove elected officials from the AHBs and to introduce new co-payments. The urgency rules were often used in Budget debates in New Zealand to introduce sales or excise tax increases (such as tobacco or gasoline tax increases) and prevent opportunistic behaviour; subsequent changes to Parliamentary procedures made urgency more difficult. Prior to the introduction of proportional representation in 1996, New Zealand's Westminster system of government could move decisively. These institutions provided an extraordinary ability to shape policy.

Other aspects of the National Government's plan required further policy development and/or legislation that could not be developed within the constraints of the Budget. Other policies were introduced in Parliament in August 1992 and later passed as the Health and Disability Services Act in March 1993 (effective on 1 July 1993), including competition between providers, the purchaser/provider split, competition between funders, portable entitlement, commercialised public hospitals, budget integration of primary and secondary care, a public health purchasing model and regional purchasing. Between 1991 and 1993, the government said that it wanted consultation on the composition of a standard benefits package and whether funding should be funded from taxes or social insurance premiums.

New co-payments and income levels for prescription medicines and for hospital services were announced and passed under urgency on the night of the 1991 Budget, and these changes took effect in February 1992.[4]

Strategies in implementation 1991–96

New Zealand's institutional structure gave ministers extraordinary leverage in developing policies, even in the absence of legislation. Officials and ministers commonly referred to the implementation of reforms in their communications. They considered the policies announced in the 1991 Budget to be in an implementation phase following the Budget, despite the lack of legislation. Health reform legislation was not introduced to Parliament until August 1992 and the Health and Disability Services Act was passed into law in March 1993, effective 1 July 1993. However, many of the critical decisions shaping the health arena were made not after 1993, but between 1991 and 1993, as new organisations and new roles in the health sector were established. Whereas implementation is commonly considered to be the process by which policy objectives get subverted, the process in New Zealand saw implementation become the arena for policy development. This section reviews the development and implementation of policy between 1991 and 1996 in terms of the perception of the policies in the public arena, and the official strategies used to manage these perceptions.

Perceptions of policies

There is considerable evidence that the public received National's 1991 Budget plans poorly and, as the next section shows, these perceptions influenced the policy development and implementation processes and corresponding policy strategies used by government. By late 1993, when government had hoped to have a system of managed competition operating, even officials considered the reform 'half-finished' as a result of 'reluctant health professionals' and 'poor public perception' (Ministry of Health, 1993f). Focus groups conducted by the government's public relations advisers showed a largely negative perception of the reforms and scepticism about the future gains. When asked if they agreed that 'health care will be more readily available', that 'more health for our money, not just more money', was required to solve problems in the health system, and whether

---

4. Co-payments were introduced partly to discourage use of hospitals over primary care doctors who cost the State less.

'the health system will be more responsive to community needs', only one third agreed (Atkinson, 1994). Whereas the government considered improved public health and a shift away from hospitals to be the future gains of reform, voters disagreed with statements such as 'by seeking to prevent illness we will all be healthier' and, finally, 'it is health care, not hospitals, that counts'. Confidence in the health care system decreased and 70 per cent of respondents had less confidence in the health system than five years previously (Atkinson, 1994). In November 1991, a poll found that 85 per cent of eligible voters disapproved of the government's handling of health issues. Women, and those aged 40–54, were the least supportive of the government's handling of health issues (Heylen/TVNZ Poll Heylen/ TVNZ, 1991). The causes of this public reaction are explored below.

First, the government's strategy of rapidly introducing health care reform through the July 1991 Budget, and especially the abolition of local representation, backfired. This strategy negatively influenced the introduction of unrelated policies, and haunted the government politically. Second, the overall public perception was that government was intent on shrinking the welfare state and privatising the health care system. This perception was helped by well organised public hospital staff, who emphasised the threat of privatisation in their communication with the press. In addition, although the espoused objective changed, at the start of the reform process ministers and officials were candid about generating fiscal savings through cuts in expenditure. Reduced expenditure was to be achieved through redefining the role and responsibility of the state for the distribution of income and provision of these services (National Archives, c1991). Once the unpopularity of reducing the scope of government became obvious, this objective was downplayed in public statements.

The public associated health reforms with a package of welfare state reforms. The government announced health and welfare reform together in December 1990. Later, in the July 1991 Budget, new welfare policies were introduced. This contributed to the public's tendency to link the health reforms to decreased state support for health funding. The government introduced both plans simultaneously and stressed the need to link entitlements for all services. The announcement of health and welfare reform united diverse groups who were able to focus on the faults of the package as a whole, and link health changes to reductions of financial support for vulnerable groups.

The policies for a commercialised hospital sector were largely based on a template used in the 1980s by Labour to restructure state industries. Not surprisingly, the public connected health reforms to economic reforms, especially in rural areas. Rural residents' incomes had been reduced and former government services (bank, postal, and rail) reduced or privatised. Commercialisation of the postal service in the 1980s had closed many post offices, much to the consternation of many rural residents.[5] Local hospitals were perceived as the final rallying point for rural people, despite the fact that many hospitals were able to provide few services. These hospitals were seen as institutions crucial for the survival of the community (Orr, 1997).

Finally, the legacy of the economic reforms of the 1980s was hostility to the idea of change itself, and a status quo bias on the part of the public. Commentators suggested the public might have developed 'battle fatigue', from successive reforms in every area of public life by 1991. This was borne out by the government's own research. One report on focus groups conducted with women in 1993 said 'there had been so many reforms in recent years that it was hard to "take in" any more' (Ministry of Health, 1993g). The period between 1991 and 1992, when the government was hoping to introduce reform, also coincided with a sharp recession. This may have made voters less willing to support market-based policies in either the economy or the welfare state. It also reduced the level of trust, since many reforms in the 1980s had paid little attention to public opinion: 'There seems to be a general distrust about anything the government does, which reflects in the highly cynical and sceptical attitude about whether the reforms would bring an improved health service. Some women were hostile about, and suspicious toward, the changes' (Ministry of Health, 1993g).

Government strategies

The government was well aware of the public perceptions of reform. Officials and ministers considered they needed to fight the perception that the reforms constituted an Americanisation of the New Zealand health care system (Ministry of Health Files, 1992e). They knew that the government's agenda was being perceived as privatisation (Ministry of Health Files, 1992i), and that the public believed a two-tier health system would result (Ministry of Health Files, 1992e). Officials firmly believed that the benefits of health care reform could be demonstrated in terms of integrated care

---

5. Rural residents did not actually lose postal services as agencies were created, but many felt attached to the local post offices that also offered banking services.

Table 5. Political and policy strategies, 1991–93

Type of opposition	Government strategy
Opposition by elected board members	Introduce legislation under urgency
Unfavourable attitudes to reform	Advertising campaign
User charges	Change rules
Legislator/National party concern over reforms	Reassurance at special conference for Cabinet, communication campaign.
Private insurance vouchers	Abandonment
Concern over level of health pending	Funds for regional health authorities held constant for 1993.
Reform concerns among public	Seminars on reforms held throughout the country.
Hospital closures	Hospitals rescued; special funds allocated.
General opposition	Implementation: policies with greatest gains introduced first.

and the benefits of separation of provider and purchaser functions, with a right to join private health care plans (Ministry of Health Files, 1992e). In response to the negative perceptions, government officials and Cabinet ministers used a number of strategies to deflect public sentiment and to reduce the potential electoral impact of the reforms. These strategies included communication and advertising campaigns (Atkinson, 1994), sequencing the implementation of reform to influence public perceptions, and manipulation of the speed of reform. Several major modifications were also made to reform policies.

Government used the media and advertising to counteract public opposition from the beginning. The political vulnerability of reform was identified as early as January 1992 (Ministry of Health Files, 1992e). In early 1991, the Minister of Health said he was keen to produce speeches, press statements and parliamentary questions that would illustrate the need for reform (Ministry of Health Files, 1991), and these efforts intensified in 1992. Government used focus groups between 1992 and 1994 to try to convince voters of the merits of reform. New Zealand reformers took note of the advice given by National Health Service reformers in the United Kingdom, who suggested that UK reforms could have been undertaken more quickly had a communications strategy been developed that informed affected groups (Ministry of Health, c1992). Therefore it became a key part of the reform process that:

A communications strategy should underpin, and be integrated with, all of the key steps in the reform process. The personal stake in health issues held by the public, the association of the health reforms with the part charging regime [co-payments], the perception of minimal action on implementation since the Budget announcements, and the complexity of the reform structures, all indicate that the reforms, to be implemented effectively, must be carefully worked through and be perceived to be soundly based and well managed. The communication and implementation process cannot be readily separated (Ministry of Health, 1991a).

The government also used five other strategies to ensure reform goals were met and to increase public support. First, the government attempted to influence the timing and the speed of reform legislation, most importantly the changes to AHBs, but later legislation as well. Bureaucrats recommended that legislation should be introduced quickly to ensure that it would be passed. They warned that any delay in the legislative process would have negative consequences (Ministry of Health, 1991d).

Second, the government used implementation sequence as a tool to affect public perceptions, after being concerned about the long lag in efficiency gains.[6] Officials thought RHAs should be introduced prior to more controversial aspects of the reforms for 'communications related reasons' (Ministry of Health, 1991a). Advisers suggested that 'changes with the greatest potential for gains should take place early, and cause users the least disruption consistent with achieving the reform objectives' (Ministry of Health, n.d.-a). Energy was therefore directed to areas where there would be positive gains in public perception, such as establishing the RHAs to purchase services for regions. RHAs were considered the 'major indicator to the public of a new reformed health service', and attention was focused on making them work (Ministry of Health, 1992e). RHAs were also considered to be 'the principal reform agencies representing the

---

6. The Minister of Health was concerned that the reforms would take a long time to generate measurable efficiency gains.

public interest' (Ministry of Health Files, 1992b).

Efforts to make RHAs the focus of 'major professional and public interests' (Ministry of Health Files, 1992b) were not successful. Given the symbolic power of hospital and (later) AHBs seen in other chapters, it is not surprising that RHAs were overshadowed by Crown Health Enterprises (CHEs). CHEs were basically twenty-three organisational units that contained former hospital board or AHB hospitals, although sometimes former boards were broken up to encourage competition within a geographic area. The Health and Disability Services Act vested ownership in the Minister for Crown Health Enterprises and the Minister of Finance, and established a number of requirements for CHEs.[7] Communities seemed to focus their negative and positive attention on these new profit-driven organisations (which were closer to the public and long established, even if under different names). CHEs received considerably more media coverage than RHAs, and RHAs received more positive or neutral media coverage (Ministry of Health, 1993d). RHAs were also associated with such issues as increased hospital charges; organisations charged with establishing the RHAs therefore suggested that decisions on user charges should be separated (Ministry of Health, 1992i).

A third strategy was to slow implementation to minimise impact. In late 1992, some ministers suggested the government should adopt a 'go slow' strategy (Ministry of Health, 1992d). Regional purchasing plans were changed in October 1992 and draft purchase plans were proposed that would 'minimally disrupt services'. Funding and service plans were left unchanged and the Minister of Health suggested that the budgets should stay the same rather than be reduced (Ministry of Health Files, 1992h). As the election neared in 1993, the government further slowed the pace of change, and officials admitted that implementation was slowing in anticipation of the election (Ministry of Health, 1993e), stating that there were 'political requirements for low impact and other factors' contributing to the difficulties. The tone of the reforms was softened: 'it became increasingly apparent that the purchaser–provider split was less about competition [substantially abandoned with health care plans] than

---

7. The legislation required CHEs to provide health care and/or disability services, and to provide the government shareholders with statements of intent while operating as a successful and efficient business to a level comparable to businesses not owned by the state. CHEs were also required to exhibit a sense of social responsibility by having regard to the interests of the communities in which they operated, to uphold ethical standards, and to be good employers.

enabling better priority setting, resource direction and rationalisation of assets and services' (Ferguson, 1995, p.193). And in 1993 the development of policy guidelines for the RHAs was affected by the need for 'fire-fighting' related to the election (Ministry of Health, 1993c). The project to develop guidelines for purchasers was also hindered by lack of political decisions and the upcoming election (Ministry of Health, 1993c).

Fourth, ministers altered the aims of policies as they were implemented. This was notable in the hospital sector, where requirements for competition and commercial approaches were frequently modified for CHEs. The transformation from public hospitals to profit-making businesses was difficult. Chief executives of CHEs admitted they found their task difficult due to high initial expectations and the reluctant public acceptance of health reform and CHE commercial roles (Ministry of Health, 1993b).

The new system was designed to reduce the ambiguities of the previous system by making government an owner or shareholder of hospitals. Instead, the new policy increased the incentives for politicians to be involved with the affairs of local hospitals. Frequent intervention by ministers ran counter to the rationale for commercialisation, which was precisely to 'let the managers manage' to ensure efficient decisions. In reality, compared to other State-Owned Enterprises (SOEs) at the time, ministers were less politically neutral. They could not let hospitals go bankrupt because of the political costs. Likewise, protests by rural residents made the fully commercial vision difficult to follow through and the government had to rescue many CHEs.

CHEs began operation with aggregate deficits of $240 million (Steering Group on the Implementation of the Coalition Agreement, 1997). Staff costs increased by 10 per cent between 1993/94 and 1995/96. The government later admitted that containing health funding was difficult due to a failure 'by the centre, to hold RHAs and CHEs accountable for achieving cost/ expenditure control' (Ministry of Health, 1996). Their public image and community resistance towards Crown Health Enterprises were considered as factors that affected CHEs' ability to borrow from the private sector (Ministry of Health, 1993a).

The uncertainties and difficulties of the new model also served to provide opportunities for the new CHEs. The new hospital organisations exploited the government's political weaknesses on hospital policy, which may have further negatively influenced the separation of social and commercial objectives. Designers of the new system hoped that the designation of the new Minister for Crown Health Enterprises would make the social and commercial objectives explicit but also separate. However, the separation was largely illusory. CHE executives admitted that they frequently targeted the Minister of Health rather than the shareholding minister when they wanted concessions on policy (Ministry of Health, 1993e).[8]

Finally, ministers abandoned or modified key policies when they were not politically popular. This was most notable in the financing area of the health reforms. Prime Minister Jim Bolger considered a competitive insurance market 'to have merits over Government monopoly of purchasing' (Ministry of Health Files, 1992f). However, in May 1992 the government decided that alternative health care plans were not part of the initial reforms and the Prime Minister in particular indicated he wanted to see the health care plans deferred into the future (Ministry of Health Files, 1992f). Competition at the financing level was not included in the implementation of health reform as ministers realised during 1992 and 1993 that the reforms were largely unpopular, making radical change considerably less favourable.

Government modified its controversial co-payment and means-testing policy. The logic was to standardise co-payment levels across services. Before 1992, doctor visits were more expensive than hospital emergency room visits for patients, which were free of charge. Primary care consultation fees had been rising much faster than the rate of inflation, by as much as 6–7 per cent per year (Ministry of Health, 1992f). In the first year, the minister received almost one thousand letters about the income classifications and co-payments (Ministry of Health).[9] Providers' experiences also influenced the survival of the policy, and public hospital staff said the public was confused and ignorant of the public hospital charging policies.

The public generally directed their disapproval and anger at the government rather than at hospital boards. Providers suggested that the elderly were described as 'bewildered' by the charges and many of the were 'in tears at the thought of having to pay' (Ministry of Health, n.d.-b). Hospitals varied in their collection of patient charges, with variation occurring from 9 to 59 per cent. Around one third (34.97 per cent) of hospital patient charges between February and August 1992 were not paid (Ministry of Health).

---

8. Officials stated that there were 'political requirements for low impact and other factors' contributing to the difficulties.
9. Refers to the number of letters in response to an Official Information Request. Various other files contain large numbers of letters regarding the health reforms in general, such as file Ministry of Health HC 29-01-1.

Government officials advised against changing the system of co-payments and means-testing since their financial estimates had not anticipated changes to the scheme (National Archives, 1991a). Officials said they were concerned about the ability for user charges to be politically influenced (Ministry of Health Files, 1992d). Treasury was against making further changes to the means-testing policies, as these would erode credibility and reduce the ability of the government to increase efficiency and expenditure; they could also create more demand for change (Ministry of Health Files, 1992g). Officials advised the minister not to modify the targeting regime because modifications would serve to 'fan public debate on its necessity' (Ministry of Health Files, 1992j), but one way to deflect this debate was devolution of user charges, which would reduce political interference (Ministry of Health Files, 1992d).

Between 1992 and 1993, many changes to the co-payment and targeting regime were made. The Minister of Health said he did not wish the new scheme of targeting and co-payments to generate 'losers' in 1993 (the election year) (Ministry of Health Files, 1992c). A new dollar stop-loss for pharmaceutical products (Ministry of Health Files, 1992a), changes to high-use benefits, a new subsidy for health care of higher-income children, and students' eligibility criteria were introduced. Maternity and accident treatment were exempted from charges, and imaging and laboratory benefits were reinstated (Ministry of Health, 1992g; Ministry of Health Files, 1992j).

A central aspect of the reforms was the establishment of a standard benefits package, for which the Core Services Committee created by the government was responsible. Like the notion of competing health care plans, this policy area was abandoned. Instead, the government pursued a more politically neutral strategy of encouraging the Core Services Committee to develop priority criteria and make recommendations about the allocation of resources. Initial expectations about the ease of this process proved overly optimistic. Early on, in September 1991, officials thought that they would shape the initial public debate on core services with an explicit package developed by 30 September 1992 (Ministry of Health, 1991g). As early as 1993, the Core Services Committee had decided against developing a list approach to defining core services. Officials were candid about the 'risks' associated with defining the core, or the risk of controversy: 'Each step in the process may become a focus for advocates of particular services, or styles of service delivery, and may not fulfil the expectation of all who have participated in the Committee's consultation and submission process'

(Ministry of Health Files, 1992b). By 1996, the committee established to define a standard benefits package had changed its name to the National Health Committee and developed a different mission (National Advisory Committee on Health and Disabilities, 1996).

In July 1992, the government appeared to reach a crisis point in the reform process: Cabinet asked officials to investigate the development of a communications and issues management strategy for the health reforms (Ministry of Health, 1992h). Discontent among backbench MPs increased throughout that year, and a seminar was specifically organised so that the Minister of Health could inform backbenchers about the implementation of the reforms and, in particular, 'manage the 'political risk' (Ministry of Health). The Health Sector Reform Management Unit was created to give the health sector stronger leadership from Wellington 'because of a hiatus and problems in the implementation process' (Ministry of Health, 1993b) and because the 'checks and balances of contestability and widespread reliable information and systems do not yet exist' (Ministry of Health, 1993b). This organisation would ensure the reforms were implemented quickly to 'drive the completion of the reform process across the health sector.' The unit would also 'provide direction to the strategic planning process by identifying the gaps and managing the potential risks' (Ministry of Health Files, 1993).

These efforts to influence the perception of health reforms through strategies of modification and reform sequencing largely failed. In 1990, 38 per cent of voters considered National's policies on health to be closest to their own views on health policy, but by 1993, just 11 per cent considered National to be closest (Table 6). The state of the health care system was a significant issue in the 1993 election, which prompted some adjustments to the policies following the election. National voters supported more expenditure on health care by government. While only 58 per cent of National voters surveyed in pre-election surveys agreed there should be free health care for all, 66 per cent considered there should be more expenditure, 31 per cent considered it should stay the same and only 3 per cent favoured less government spending on health care (Vowles and Aimer, 1993). Only 21 per cent of National voters agreed there should be a reduction in taxation for health and education expenditure (Vowles and Aimer, 1993).

Table 6. Party positions on health: alignment with voters' views 1990–96: which is closest to your own position on health?[10]

(%)	1990**	1993	1996
National	38.6	11.1	12.5
All other parties*	41.5	73.4	77.1
I don't know	14.5	15.7	10.5

* In 1993 this included categories such as 'none' and 'multiple parties'.
** In 1990 voters were given an option of 'no difference between National and Labour' and 20.5 per cent chose this option in 1990.

The 1993 election also contained a constitutional referendum on the electoral system. However, National was unable to restore public confidence in health care reform. Surveys undertaken from 1993 to 1996 showed that the public had unfavourable views of the National Party's ability to improve the health system. The public consistently favoured the Labour Party as the party that was thought most able to improve the health system, and other parties such as the left-wing Alliance and New Zealand First also received support for their policies (UMR Insight, 1993–1996b).

By the end of 1994, almost three quarters of voters considered the reforms a failure, with just 10 per cent of voters considering them a success. Health reforms received the most support from National voters, but this support was still low (16 per cent). Most National voters considered the reforms a failure (59 per cent of National voters) (UMR Insight, 1993–1996a).

The survival of policies in the late 1990s

The health care system envisaged by the Minister of Health in 1991 assumed that purchasers in the public and private sectors would assume the roles of AHBs. Regional purchasers (including insurance companies) would be required to purchase services mandated by a nationally established

---

10. In 1990, voters were asked which of the two main parties' views on these issues came closest to their own views on each issue. National and Labour were the only party options in 1990. No Difference was not given as an option after 1990. None was given as an option only in 1996.

standard benefits package, and competition would introduce discipline. This package of policies shifted dramatically between 1991 and 1997 (Table 7) and many of National's 1991 proposals became undone.

National entered the 1996 election campaign with a disadvantage, as health was a major concern of voters who firmly associated the poor state of the public health system with the National governments of 1990 and 1993. New Zealand First had campaigned on a platform of populist policies and had expressed opposition to National Party policy, including health policy. In December 1996, a National–New Zealand First Coalition Government was formed. In 1997, the Government reviewed health policies and made some fundamental changes, discussed in more detail in the next chapter. Electoral law changes[11] and the necessity that National cooperate with other parties to form a government largely prompted the Government's 1997 review.

The National–New Zealand First Coalition proposed a number of changes to the health system that were outlined in the Coalition Agreement.[12] The Agreement on Health expanded health care access and reduced co-payments and means testing. Funding for health was increased, doctor visits for all children under six became free, all user charges for hospitals were removed, and waiting list/waiting time funds were increased. In a 1997 review of the 1990s health reforms, the government admitted that the public had harboured fears about obtaining access to health services and concerns about service quality (Steering Group on the Implementation of the Coalition Agreement, 1997). Many features of the health care system that were implemented were shown as ineffective. Government-owned health care facilities failed to deliver efficiency savings through competitive contracting. RHAs were unable to provide access to health care that was demanded by funding contracts. Both the public and clinicians expressed concerns about the profit objectives of CHEs (Steering Group on the

11. In 1996, electoral reform had the outcome that the election was held under proportional representation rules.

12. The agreement stated that it would centralise the RHAs, provide free doctor visits for children under six, remove the requirement for hospitals to be profitable, increase allocations to a fund designed to reduce waiting times for operations, remove asset testing for long-term care, review the health sector as a whole, abolish hospital co-payments, develop Māori health initiatives, increase health funding, create criteria for private sector involvement in 'services usually provided by the public service', rationalise ministerial portfolios, and re-consider funding arrangements for accident victims.

Implementation of the Coalition Agreement, 1997).

Regional purchasing underwent a number of modifications. As noted above, in the first year (1992 to 1993) purchasers were instructed to obtain the same services they had in 1991 (New Zealand Department of Health, 1992). Government's regional purchaser roles shifted through the implementation process. RHAs changed to become non-commercial

Table 7. 1991 survival of policies

Ministerial proposal 1991	Implementation process	Survival
Competition between Providers	Moderated: not pure competition model – central co-ordination	Mixed
Co-payments	Charges introduced in 1991 to 1992. Laboratory charges dropped; in-patient hospital charges dropped. Primary and Pharmaceutical charges remained. Hospital and in-patient charges dropped in 1996.	No
Standard Benefits Package – 'Core' Services	Abandoned approx. 1994. Replaced with emphasis on priority setting, development of guidelines, and developing notion of access based on clinical criteria.	No
Competition between Regional Health Authorities	Not implemented	No
Profit requirements for public hospitals	Abandoned approx. 1996–97	No
Regional purchasing	Lasted until 1996 then centralised: now one Health Funding Authority.	No
Opt-out provision and vouchers for health insurance	Not implemented	No
Limit government funding for health services to the neediest	Some universal health benefits introduced in 1997, means-testing remains for many other services. However, state remains dominant health funder.	No
Purchaser–provider split for hospital services	Implemented and moderated somewhat in 1996 to 1999.	Yes
Elected members of Area Health Boards	Immediately introduced in July 1991. All board members fired.	Yes

institutions designed to be responsive to the community. By May 1992, the Minister of Health instructed officials that RHAs should not be 'seen as fully commercial enterprises' and that more community consultation and community involvement was necessary (Ministry of Health, 1991e, Ministry of Health, 1992a). RHAs did not compete for customers but retained responsibility for residents within their area. RHAs were finally abandoned in 1996 in favour of a single purchasing agency with small regional offices.

The RHAs were designed in the context of two other policies that were also abandoned. Reformers assumed that health authorities would be facing competition from private health insurers that would make contracts to provide a set of core services for individuals. Negotiations between ministers and public servants revealed that policy development on RHAs was based on an assumption that there would be competition in the market and that RHAs would also be constrained by mandated 'core' health services funded by social insurance premiums that would be levied on all families.[13] The main aim of the core services plan was to enable monitoring of purchasing organisations to ensure that individuals enrolled with insurers were receiving the care offered in the plan. Specification of benefits would make it easier to monitor RHA performance, because individuals would be able to alert government to deficiencies of RHA provision through the political process (Ministry of Health, 1992b). Without a standard benefits package, regulating RHAs was more difficult. The lack of a benefits package also raised questions about how to determine the best balance between commercial and social objectives. Originally the RHAs would have a clear commercial mandate that would give managers the right incentives, and protect them from political interference (Ministry of Health, 1992c).

As discussed above, in the hospital sector alterations to reform plans were made in many areas, despite initial success in removing elected officials. After the government removed elected members of AHBs, it gained more control over the hospital sector. However, the business model proposed for hospitals and intended to provide incentives to keep institutions efficient

---

13. Premiums would be adjusted for risk factors such as family size, age and gender. Future adjustments for lifestyle factors were anticipated to encourage economic use of health services. Premiums would be paid for all children. The per capita cost of premiums for those receiving no assistance from government was estimated at NZ$650–2220 per year. Couples with two children would pay part of their premium at incomes of around $35,000 per year, and those earning $40,000 and above would pay the full cost of their premiums. Premiums would be capped at $1250, $1500 or $2000 per annum.

was not successful (National Interim Provider Board, 1992).

By 1996, a review of the reforms suggested health should be moved further away from the model of competition and stressed the value of a long-term focus, collaborative and constructive relationships, outcome-based services, transparent rationing, and culturally appropriate services. Participation was espoused as a central value: 'Communities have the right to participate, and funders and providers are responsible for ensuring communities' values and preferences are reflected in decision-making' (Steering Group on the Implementation of the Coalition Agreement, 1997, p.11). These kinds of recommendations stand in stark contrast to the values espoused in the 1991 report 'Your Health and the Public Health', which envisioned efficiency through competition.

The government implied that the reforms had failed to meet cost containment objectives. Government contributed a smaller proportion of total health care expenditure but found it difficult to contain the rate of growth in the public sector. Since 1993, there had been frequent ad hoc allocations to the health budget that resulted in an average annual growth rate of 1.9 per cent per capita (real), excluding transfers and capital. Between 1996 and 1997, ad hoc additions to health accounted for over 11 per cent of the total health budget (Ministry of Health, 1996).

Conclusion

The perceptions and strategies of both the public and politicians were shown through the period discussed in this chapter as a significant factor that influenced the development and implementation of policy reform in the 1990s. The National Government of 1990 entered office with bold plans to reform the welfare state and to transfer many state functions to the private sector. Between December 1990 and July 1991, officials quickly developed a plan for the health sector that would break up AHBs into competing hospitals. Purchasers would receive funding from government or private insurers. A mandated standard benefit package would regulate purchasers and provide the package of services within which purchasers and insurers would develop contracts with providers. In July 1991, the government quickly introduced Budget legislation to eliminate the power of AHBs, the same institutions that had effectively prevented major reform over the past century. The government also moved quickly to introduce new co-payments and means tests and then set to work to further develop other aspects of the reform plan.

Hospital boards had been the most troublesome feature of health care reform during the twentieth century. However, once boards were no longer localised (after 1989) or representative (after 1991), the government faced new opposition to radical policy reform. Westminster institutional structures at first appeared to facilitate 'easy' reform but the actual outcome of health care reform in its implementation showed considerable deviations from the plans announced in 1991. The public was not in favour of the sweeping reform proposals, as demonstrated by numerous polls and focus groups. The government's earlier claims that it would reduce the role of the state and re-orient the welfare state did not help the popularity of reform. The public, in particular, feared that New Zealand would follow the United States. Finally, after seven years of reform under Labour during the 1980s, the public was growing resistant to change. Public perception was significant in the implementation of reforms.

In response to the unpopularity of the reforms, the government adopted five main strategies. Ministers used communication campaigns to persuade the public of the merits of reform, and introduced legislation quickly. Ministers timed the sequence and direction of implementation, slowed the implementation of some policies, altered the aims of many policies and abandoned some altogether. Between 1992 and 1993, numerous modifications were made to the model of health reform, as political necessities prompted reconsideration. Ministers faced abundant incentives to dilute their plans.

The perceptions of the public and the strategies of politicians have fundamental consequences for the design and implementation of policies. On this occasion, the government failed to fully implement the internal market, which resulted in a quasi-internal market that assumed competitive purchasing and portable financing on the part of individuals, overlaid on a system designed for an earlier age of area hospital-based grants. 'Mimic markets' or competition within the framework of services that continue to be publicly managed and financed present a peculiar hybrid, as Rudolf Klein has observed (Klein, 1996). In New Zealand, as in Britain, this largely unintended hybrid model had fundamental implications for the successful operation of the health care system. The system that emerged represented political compromises rather than technocratic blueprints for efficiency.

By 1996, electoral incentives operating in the new proportional representation system conspired to put National in office with one of the parties opposing its health care reforms, New Zealand First. New electoral rules enabled new parties to capture disenchanted voters and the new National–New Zealand First Coalition Government introduced a number of changes to the health system that further modified National's plans.

Health care reform in New Zealand between 1990 and 1996 shows the primacy of political institutions for understanding policy. The analysis of reform confirms that, without Westminster institutions, politicians would not contemplate such sweeping reforms. Nor would politicians have been able to overturn one hundred years of local representation. Changing political institutions (the electoral system and thus the party relationships in New Zealand government) served to bring in new interests to the Cabinet table after 1996, which also fundamentally influenced health policy.

However, the possibilities of Westminster institutions also created limitations. The National Government thought that if political representation in the health care system was overturned, reform might be less troublesome. But the removal of the AHBs destroyed a buffer between government and the public that ultimately cost the government many of its policy reforms. The institutions of government served to focus the blame (Weaver, 1986) for problems arising from reform implementation on where power lay (the Minister of Health and Cabinet). Thus, while these political institutions ultimately gave politicians the ability to introduce radical policies, they did not provide the means to realise their policy goals once the costs and benefits were clear to electors.

CHAPTER SEVEN

The rise and demise of the Health Funding Authority

A T THE 1993 general election, following several years of discussion and debate about New Zealand's electoral system, the public was presented with options for electoral system reform on which to vote. The result was a move to proportional representation. The next election, in 1996, was the first conducted under the new Mixed Member Proportional (MMP) electoral system, which has since produced a series of coalition governments. The post-election formation of the inaugural 1996 coalition government followed protracted discussions between the New Zealand First Party, who held the balance of power, and each of the two main political parties, National and Labour, each with similar levels of voter support. The result was a coalition of the New Zealand First and National parties that included a number of new policy agreements hammered out between them. A core part of these was a reconfiguration of the 1993 health reforms, commencing another period of health sector change. The new directions included removing the for-profit focus from public hospital services, centralising purchasing functions, and emphasising health outcomes. While the new directions reflected several New Zealand First Party aims, the formation of the coalition government also provided an opportunity to deal with some of the problems created by the 1993 health reforms, and to further some of the directions which the National Government had begun to emphasise in response to some of the failures of health reforms outlined in the previous chapter (Shipley, 1995).[1]

---

1. Parts of this chapter draw upon discussions in Gauld (2009).

The period discussed in this chapter (1996–2000) saw the establishment of the national Health Funding Authority (HFA) as purchaser, replacing the RHAs. The HFA era, which spanned only one three-year electoral cycle, was marked by a series of different policy directions. Some were remnants from the prior era of competition, others signified a new set of political and health system objectives. The goals and direction of the health system continued to evolve through the period, along with the changes taking place. The years 1997 and 1998 were a time of uncertainty, as the new system was under construction. From 1999, with the HFA 'up and running', the focus was on consolidating the changes and working towards nationally consistent purchasing and service delivery frameworks.

The HFA era was short but complex for a variety of reasons. Foremost was the fact that this was a period of considerable change, but also of continuity. The coalition government appeared to be committed to a different focus for health policy and a series of new emphases emerged. However, commitment to a number of the core principles from the 1993–96 health reforms era was evident until at least early 1999 and, indeed, the subsequent Labour-led Coalition Government (discussed in the next chapter) highlighted, in its pre-election campaigning, a need to reverse the policy emphasis on provider competition and rejuvenate the role of the public in governance and decision-making. In terms of governance, the HFA period might be described as one in which there were gradual moves towards engaging communities in the decision-making process, albeit via a centrally controlled set of structures that featured appointee-only hospital boards. In this respect, the period confirmed the policy of corporate-style governance and was, again, an historical deviation. The HFA era was also marked by the disintegration of the coalition government eighteen months after its formation, with the National Party retaining its grip on power. While New Zealand First had provided pressure for new directions, the coalition breakup made way for National to dominate health policy once again. Finally, a hallmark of the HFA era was so-called 'sector-led' policy (Creech, 1999), which effectively meant government looked to providers, health professionals and communities to both initiate health policy ideas and to provide advice and feedback to government on policy issues. Thus, there was a level of engagement not evident in the prior competitive period of the early 1990s. While this indicated an attempt to reach out to the public and health sector, such engagement occurred within a centralised and controlled infrastructure and, in this way, was a model of top-down control.

This chapter considers the changes to organisational configuration, the key policy initiatives, and the primary gains of the period from the 1996 election to beyond the 1999 election, which produced a Labour–Alliance Coalition Government. Although the Labour-led Coalition introduced a new round of health restructurings (detailed in the next chapter), the existing structures and programmes remained in place in the interim. Some of these would be retained, others gradually phased out.

The 'Coalition Agreement on Health'

The National–New Zealand First Coalition Government 'Coalition Agreement on Health' contained a set of new principles for health policy development, along with a series of new policy initiatives. Underpinning the coalition's policies were concerns that relationships and performance across the health sector remained ineffective, that providers (including the health workforce) failed to see the relevance of the competitive environment, that the public lacked confidence in the health system, that the contracting system had proved costly to administer, and that the system lacked coordination or strategic direction (Ministry of Health, 1996a; Steering Group, 1997). These were issues that different advisers, including the Treasury, Ministry of Health and the Crown Company Monitoring Advisory Unit (CCMAU) had highlighted in their 1996 briefings to the incoming government. Each provided a different perspective on the health system.

The Treasury made note of the gains from the prior competitive era, including hospital throughput increases of 4 per cent, a rise from 65 to 80 per cent in immunisation rates, declining growth rates in pharmaceutical expenditure, improved access to Māori health services, and introduction of capitation and budget-holding for primary care 'with positive results' (Treasury, 1996, p.99). But the Treasury also highlighted various problems, such as expanding waiting lists and times, and disparities in health outcomes among different groups – with Māori and Pacific Islanders most affected – across a range of indicators, including infant mortality, immunisation rates and lifestyle-related conditions. On the competitive structures themselves, Regional Health Authorities (RHAs) and Crown Health Enterprises (CHEs), Treasury suggested the benefits of change could take '4 to 8 years to work through' (Treasury, 1996, p.101). Initial results showed that purchasers 'overspent' budgets, while central government intervened in decision-making. CHEs had failed to produce expected gains: only Pharmac (Pharmaceutical Management Agency of New Zealand) made 'significant savings'. Treasury's advice was to improve accountabilities (perhaps through a reward system), be clear about the limited resource base and need for rationing, let structures evolve over time through encouraging 'bottom-up' innovations, commit to budgets and devolve responsibilities for these, and strive for cooperation with clinicians as they had 'significant influence in promoting best cost-effective practice' (Treasury, 1996, p.102). Advice from the Ministry of Health broadly mirrored that of Treasury. Implicit was the belief that structural change was needed. Thus, the Ministry provided a list of 'desirable features' for any new arrangements, including service integration, responsiveness to patients, directing of resources to priority areas, clinical involvement in resource allocation, and reduced hospital domination (Ministry of Health, 1996a). However, while officials were an important source of advice to the government, the Coalition Agreement on Health was essentially the result of negotiations between the coalition partners.

The Agreement listed principles for health policy and public services delivery that were considered to be 'non-negotiable.' These included retaining the purchaser–provider split, maintaining the 'business-like' focus of the sector while emphasising health improvement in purchasing and planning processes, and continuing to develop monitoring, audit and information systems to enhance financial accountability. The major changes presided over by the National–New Zealand First Coalition were:

- Combining the four RHAs into a single national funding body, the HFA, which was to focus on promoting collaboration rather than competition amongst providers. Collaboration was to be promoted through shifting the contracting process away from competitive tendering, which was the focus under the RHAs, to a process based on historic funding levels, benchmarking information, and comparative data – especially around costs of providing services by, and prices paid to, different providers.

- Removing the for-profit objective of health provision and replacing this with principles of 'public service', but requiring that providers continue to be 'business-like'.

- Renaming and reorienting the Crown Health Enterprises to become Hospital and Health Services (HHSs).

- Limiting private involvement in the provision of public health services and limiting government 'bureaucracy' where possible.

- Emphasising outcomes in the purchase and monitoring of health services.

- Increasing health funding to ensure that levels were 'sustainable'. This was a result of a pre-election review that found funding levels had severely stretched several CHEs and threatened patient safety (Ministry of Health, 1996b).
- Reducing elective surgery waiting times, bolstering child and mental health services, and Māori health development.
- Providing free doctor visits and prescription medicines for children aged five years and under (Coalition Agreement, 1996).

A 'Steering Group' was formed in early 1997 to advise on further development and implementation of the Coalition's policies. They would report back to the government by mid-year. In an attempt by government to involve officials more closely in policy development and implementation than had been the case with the 1993–96 reforms, the twelve-member Steering Group was chaired by the Director-General of Health at the time, Dr Karen Poutasi. The aim was to 'involve people with health and disability sector knowledge and backgrounds' (Steering Group, 1997, Appendix 1). In this regard, there was an attempt to bring institutional knowledge to the process, but also to reach out to the broader policy community and health service providers and, in this way, engender a level of participation and ownership of the new policy directions. Steering Group members were primarily funder and provider representatives from a variety of areas in the health system, such as Māori health and primary care, with an initial expectation that the group would consult widely with affected parties and agencies throughout its deliberations. However, given the short time frame allowed for the Steering Group's work, it was decided to alter its terms of reference to circumvent wide consultation and instead invite public submissions once the report had been delivered.

The Steering Group returned with a variety of recommendations that reflected the shift in health policy directions which had occurred throughout the HFA period. These recommendations confirmed the coalition's broader policy directions, including the statement that the health sector must have a long-term common strategic vision, which should be to improve the health and independence of New Zealanders. It was suggested that change should follow an evolutionary process in order to avoid the disruption and uncertainty of previous change eras. The health sector, the Steering Group noted, was clearly tired of change, with 'three reforms over the past 10 years' (Steering Group, 1997, p.59). As public confidence rested on sector confidence, the coalition's reforms should not be oversold as a panacea, but presented realistically with communication messages supporting the theme of 'evolution not revolution' (Steering Group, 1997, p.62). In tandem with this, it was asserted that there should be an emphasis on ensuring that relationships at all levels of the sector – both horizontal amongst providers and vertical between purchasers and providers – should be collaborative and cooperative. This, it was suggested, would best be promoted through seeking the participation of 'individuals, communities, health professionals and organisations' in decision-making and organisational development (Steering Group, 1997, p.7, p.10). As an example, the group suggested that to facilitate building relationships within the new HHSs (Hospital and Health Services), managers needed to involve health professionals in all management, contracting and planning processes. When it came to contracting, which remained core to the split between purchaser and providers, the report recommended that processes should be based on aligned objectives and the development of good relationships between contract partners. There would be no need for secrecy and insular behaviour among HHSs, as they no longer had to compete with one another. Instead, the focus for service providers should be on coordination and patient outcomes. The report said government needed to recognise that health status was influenced by factors often beyond the ambit of the health system. Health sector coordination would help improve health status, as would collaboration between government agencies such as housing, education, welfare and local government. Finally, the Steering Group recommended the government should be clear about the requirement for rationing and prioritisation, with processes for this to be explicit, transparent, and therefore open to public scrutiny.

The Coalition's policies and Steering Group recommendations were viewed positively by national and international observers for their promise to nurture cooperation, build relationships and restore confidence in the health system (Ham, 1997; Martin, 1997). However, subsequent developments suggested that only some elements of the coalition policies were promoted; other changes indicated attempts to repackage ideas introduced in 1993, in particular, promoting competition and core service definition, which fed into the hands of the Labour opposition in positioning itself for the 1999 election. Moreover, crucial elements of the health reforms remained, including the purchaser-provider split and service contracting. Similarly, while the policy settings changed, it was some time before the ethos of officialdom followed. In the interim – until at least 1999 – the purchasing and monitoring workforce remained committed to notions of competition, efficiency and financial accountability, with the breakup of the Coalition providing further support for this. Finally, the processes of change enacted by the Coalition Agreement commenced yet another period of dissolving institutional knowledge, as had also happened through the creation of the competitive system described in the previous chapter.

The process and politics of forming the new central purchaser

As the new central purchasing agency was created, several hangovers from the previous competitive era could be seen, suggesting deviation from the new policy directions. To commence the change process, in mid-1997 the Transitional Health Authority (THA) was created to preside over the dissolution of the four RHAs and the amalgamation of their functions into a single purchasing agency. The government appointed Graham Scott as chairperson of the THA board. Scott had been Treasury secretary under both the Labour and National governments (1986–93), was very influential in policy circles across a range of key state-sector reforms (Goldfinch, 1998), and pivotal to the development and promotion of public service 'markets' and new public management through that era (Scott et al., 1990). He had been a member of the Steering Group and, previously, an RHA chair.

Following his appointment, Scott announced that the restructurings in 1993 had failed as the government neither committed to the original design nor encouraged competition within the health sector (*Otago Daily Times*, 23 September 1997). This view was expressed in discussion papers produced for the THA, which concluded that the '[health reforms] model was troubled by implementation problems rather than fundamental design flaws' (McKenzie Webster, 1997a, p.6) and that this was the main reason why the various policy adaptations described in the previous chapter had been introduced by politicians. Significantly, around the time of the THA formation, Neil Kirton, the New Zealand First Party Associate Minister of Health, was removed from his post. Kirton had consistently charged that the National Party had no intention of adhering to the Coalition Agreement on Health and was instead harbouring a covert agenda to continue with the directions set in 1993. While the New Zealand First Leader, Winston Peters, removed Kirton for allegedly breaching an agreement not to comment in public on a series of ongoing disputes with the Minister of Health, Bill English, Kirton suggested that 'Mr Peters essentially offered me the choice of becoming a house-trained, neutered, National Party poodle, unable to effectively defend the public health system. I rejected such a total breach of the principles that elected me to Parliament and NZ First to power' (*Otago Daily Times*, 8 July 1997).

The THA's initial work involved head office and operational plan development, while also assuming all health services purchasing responsibilities (Ministry of Health, 1997), a task initially undertaken by around twenty staff. During this period, the four RHAs became regional offices of the THA. The change process undermined staff morale and all four RHA chief executives and a number of senior managers subsequently resigned. Research into the change process suggested many staff found it particularly stressful having to continue with RHA work as usual while facing an uncertain future (Gauld, 2003). It was unclear whether local offices would be retained and, if so, how many of these there would be. Many saw the move to a single purchaser as amounting to a 'takeover', and could not see the advantages of a central purchaser. Even if existing structures and offices were retained, there would be reduced autonomy, as the agencies would sit under a new layer of bureaucracy. With centralisation, the 'closeness' to providers through regional presence would be lost, as would the differing purchasing methods used by the four bodies and the capacity this provided for experimentation and inter-agency learning. Finally, the RHAs were opposed to restructuring after only three years in operation. It had taken at least the first two years from the commencement of the health reforms in mid-1993 to 'learn' about the purchaser role. With the new structure, this learning process – largely about people becoming acquainted with their roles and building working relationships – would have to start again from scratch (Gauld, 2003).

As noted above, the THA chair commissioned a series of consultant reports looking at different aspects of the service delivery environment that had developed under the RHA and CHE structures (McKenzie Webster, 1997a). The various recommendations from these reports underpinned subsequent HFA policy, as discussed below. While some of the reports provided advice for the way forward in keeping with the Coalition Agreement and Steering Group recommendations, they also noted that there was a need for change in the existing environment for purchasing and providing, and in particular that the issue of CHE deficits (or funding levels) needed to be addressed (McKenzie Webster, 1997b). In lieu of this, it was unlikely that contract negotiations would proceed with good will, good relationships were unlikely to develop, the focus would continue to be on the short term, and third-party intervention in the negotiating process would continue to be required. In short, there would be little contextual change from the RHA-CHE period.

In early 1998, an amended Health and Disability Services Act saw the Health Funding Authority (HFA) replace the THA and take responsibility for the four RHA offices. In keeping with the focus through much of the 1990s on what was considered to be the right background for high-level health sector appointments, Phil Pryke, a businessman with no prior experience in health, was appointed as HFA chief executive. The subject of some controversy, particularly over his level of remuneration, Pryke resigned after little more than a year. The HFA drew some staff from the RHAs but also selected new staff committed to the new structures and policy directions. In this respect, it remains unclear what the intent of the government and HFA management was: to forge ahead with aspects of the competitive market health reforms of 1993–96 which had remained static, to implement policy in keeping with the coalition agreement, or to pursue some form of middle-ground between these two directions.

With senior management in place, the HFA next contracted an Australian firm, LEK Consulting, to review the organisation of purchasing and develop a new national structure to replace the four RHAs. Predictably perhaps, given the policy settings of the 1993 health reforms, the LEK review found that the existing structure contained four incomparable organisations, the RHAs, and that the organisation of staff had been poorly developed and controlled. There were no clear or comparable job descriptions across the agencies and considerable overlaps between task areas. Accordingly, and in keeping with the coalition pledge to limit bureaucracy, LEK recommended the purchasing structures be completely revamped. Given the replication of work across four regional organisations, inefficiencies this involved, and the gains that could be made with single national work groups, it was anticipated that the HFA would be able to function with fewer staff than the RHAs had. Following this, in mid-1998 almost all of the HFA's 520 staff, taken on from the RHAs, were disestablished and given the option of applying for one of 370 new posts scheduled to be in place by the end of 1998 (Health Funding Authority, 1998c). Both the Ministry of Health, responsible for monitoring HFA performance, and the HFA itself raised concern at the loss of key personnel and related institutional and technical knowledge (Health Funding Authority, 1998c). While it took some time for the HFA to recover from the transition process, and it was at least the end of 1998 before the agency was fully able to focus on the purchasing task, the intent of the internal reconfiguration process was to develop an appropriate agency structure for the long term. In the interim, one of the ways in which the HFA attempted to address the problem of institutional knowledge was to define, standardise and document all work systems and processes, as would a company seeking ISO9000 certification (Health Funding Authority, 1998c). With this established, any employee would, at least in theory, be able to simply perform tasks by following instructions and guidelines.

The core functions of the HFA remained the same as the RHAs, albeit with some different expectations. Prior to the Coalition Agreement, RHAs were concerned with obtaining the greatest volumes for the money and did little to ensure that funding levels were reasonable or services safe (Stent, 1998). Following the Agreement, both contract parties were expected to work more closely to ensure that purchasing decisions were based on reliable information and, through establishing benchmark prices and further application of a population-based funding formula, that funding levels would be regionally equitable. However, in addition to getting the HFA established, the transition to collaborative contracting was subject to various setbacks.

First, the HFA set funding levels at head office, but allowed a series of locality managers to negotiate local contracts. This failed to reverse inequities in prices and purchaser expectations across different regions and implicitly reinforced competitive behaviours. Second, funding levels continued to be below the level of demand in the community. As noted above, funding increases were necessary in order to promote good relationships between contracting parties and give effect to the new directions. In the absence of a significant increase, standoffs continued to affect contract negotiations between the HFA and providers. The situation was compounded by the fact that the government and its agencies had no immediate strategy in place to fund provider deficits (or reduce underfunding), or reduce demand for services. The National Health Committee (previously Core Services Committee), whose role had been to focus on rationing, continued to focus on prioritisation at the periphery of health care delivery and produce reports on various issues. The HFA did commence a process for prioritisation of all funding decisions but this never got beyond the planning stage before the agency was disestablished. In any case, implementing the HFA's process could have proved politically difficult. It involved applying economic methods for ranking services based on contribution to health need and outcomes and would have meant certain services with lower rankings having funding withdrawn (Health Funding Authority, 1998b). In the meantime, the view that efficiency gains would mean services could be provided within available funding continued to dominate. Third, the state of flux the purchaser experienced due to the transitional process further undermined relationship-building between the contracting parties. Fourth, and in keeping with its desired policy for primary care organisation (contained in a five-year plan that would see general practitioners formally organised into 'primary health service organisations'), the HFA indicated through the contracting process its wish to move services out of hospitals and into the community (Health Funding Authority, 1998a).

To be fair, the HFA was only fully functional from the end of 1998, and Ministry of Health quarterly reports, which commenced in mid-1997, indicated regular improvements in HFA performance (Ministry of Health, 2000). From 1999 onwards, there was more clarity and a sense of purpose within and external to the HFA, and contrasts with the RHA era became more evident as further discussed in the next section. There was a concerted attempt to develop good collaborative relationships with providers through regular and ongoing contact and engagement in the planning process, although relationship problems and information-sharing difficulties remained (Ministry of Health, 1999, p.30). A major focus was on achieving nationally consistent funding and service coverage through standardised contracts and information, with an ultimate aim of developing longer-term 'evergreen' contracts. This was underpinned by the increased emphasis on using a population-based funding formula focused on patient catchment, evidence and health outcomes (rather than service cost), and public dissemination of service costing and funding information. There was also more emphasis in the planning and contracting process on enhancing service integration and health improvement. Considerable effort was put into developing nationally consistent tools for prioritising patients on waiting lists for elective surgery and developing methods to prioritise funding, although this area remained troubled (Gauld and Derrett, 2000) and has continued to be the case. A specific fund was established for promoting Māori provider development and Māori health improvement programmes, in line with Māori Health Commission advice (Māori Health Commission, 1999). There was an attempt to emphasise public health through the development of national programmes in areas such as cancer screening and tobacco control, and requiring general practitioners to focus on the health of their patients rather than on episodic treatment. Finally, the HFA engaged in forward planning through charting a 'mid- to long-term development path' (Health Funding Authority, 2000).

The HFA's focus was bolstered by the government's 'medium-term' strategy for the health sector, issued by the Minister of Health, Wyatt Creech, shortly after he replaced Bill English in early 1999 (Creech, 1999). This was a further attempt to stabilise and provide direction for the sector. The strategy, which was something of a pre-election manifesto for National, contained twelve goals. These aimed to improve services for selected groups, provide certainty to the public around issues of access and service availability, coordinate services, focus on public health and health outcomes, enhance inter-sector collaboration, achieve financial sustainability and consult the public in the planning process for key decisions.

This last aspect of the medium-term strategy, community consultation, was the key mechanism for involving the public in health-care planning and policy-making through the HFA period and, of course, during the prior years of the competitive market model. It was an area on which the National Health Committee had provided advice. In a discussion paper prepared for a THA workshop, the Committee suggested that communities sometimes needed to be informed of decisions once taken; at other times it was appropriate to seek community input as an important source of information when analysing policy options, but only as one of several sources. In many cases, particularly those where resources were being reallocated or prioritised, there would be quite different views from different public groups, meaning decision-makers would have to balance these views in reaching a final decision. What was most important, then, was to apply a consistent framework for analysis. In the New Zealand context this was that the outcome of any decision should do more good than harm, should provide value for money, should promote fairness in access and use of resources, and should be consistent with community values (National Health Committee, 1997). That said, the extent to which the HFA consulted regional services and communities remained a sore point and one the HFA sought to improve. Indeed, by 1999 it had put in place locality managers and regional offices with a clear directive to consult with local providers – at least – and to attempt to reach out to the broader community.

The Ministry of Health, for its part, remained largely untouched, at least in structural terms. That said, the agency did come under scrutiny. In theory, the HFA was accountable to the Ministry. However, having the HFA as an independent agency with direct reporting lines to the Minister of Health meant the two agencies often independently developed policy on the same issues with limited coordination or collaboration in their activities. This possibility had been highlighted in analytical work on the new structures, with suggestions that roles would have to be clearly defined (Hawkins and Vaithianathan, 1997). In recognition of this, in 1998, the Ministry of Health issued a five-year plan acknowledging the need for role definition. The plan stated that the Ministry would reduce its involvement in operational matters, with several functions being handed over to the HFA, and in future would focus on three core functions: policy advice, ministerial servicing and HFA monitoring (Ministry of Health, 1998).

Assessing the HFA period

Given the short time the HFA was in operation, any assessment of the period remains difficult, particularly as the new structures were really functional only from around 1999 and most policy issues continued to be in development. By the end of the period, there were clear signs of some gains, as noted in the *Briefing for the Incoming Government* produced by the HFA just prior to the 1999 election (Health Funding Authority, 1999). While subject to an HFA bias, the briefing attempted to compare performances with the RHA era and outlined improvements across a variety of dimensions.

In the purchasing and contracting arena, for instance, the HFA suggested there had been a clear shift toward national frameworks focused on equity, with collaboratively reached agreements aimed at service integration. The long-term plan was for a stronger focus on health outcomes, with provider networks being contracted to provide a range of integrated services within a quality improvement paradigm. On planning for service delivery, the HFA suggested it had overseen a transition from fragmented provision to an environment in which there was considerable information-sharing amongst providers and a plan that showed the public the services they were entitled to and where they could expect to receive these. Future plans were for a heightened emphasis on locality planning, with needs assessments and increased public involvement playing an important part in this. The primary care 'Independent Practitioner Associations' (further discussed in the next chapter), that had emerged through the 1990s, were ready for integrated care contracting and to lead in building stronger organisational foundations for general practice and multi-disciplinary approaches to primary care delivery. For prioritisation, the HFA suggested it had developed a robust and practicable framework for future purchasing decisions, while service access for elective surgery was routinely assessed using standardised scoring tools. However, there remained considerable inconsistency amongst HHSs in the tools used, with the result that inequities in access persisted.

The HFA suggested that under the RHAs there had been twenty-three Māori health providers. Through focused planning and the creation of a strong Māori health team, the agency had facilitated growth to over 200 Māori providers, with a future plan for specific Māori health targets and integrated Māori health organisations. In the area of pharmaceuticals, the HFA reported that Pharmac (the government's independent drug-buying agency) had slowed growth in expenditure to about 3 per cent per annum, down from about 10 per cent under the RHAs. Future plans included increased emphasis on demand-side strategies. Finally, the HFA argued that several advances had been made in public health, including development of national cancer screening and tobacco control programmes, and an emphasis on public health throughout the sector, especially in primary care settings, with plans to further focus providers on public health following the 1999 election.

Conclusion: another election, another health system

By the time of the 1999 general election, it appeared that the HFA system was beginning to show promise and there was a reasonably clear plan – at least from the HFA's perspective – for the way ahead. The purchasing structure was maturing and new policy programmes, such as those for more integrated primary care delivery, were under way. There seemed to be an effort to build nationally consistent service delivery arrangements. The financial environment for hospitals was showing signs of improvement, independent practitioner associations were in a strong position to lead a more robust primary care sector, and the Ministry of Health was settling into its role of strategic policy advice and HFA monitoring. Furthermore, there had been significant Māori health organisational gains, an increased focus on public health, and work was in process to increase the level of community involvement in planning and decision-making. However, an array of problems remained, as may be expected with a newly created set of arrangements, and public confidence in the health system was low (Donelan et al., 1999). With National having occupied the Treasury benches for three electoral terms, the public voted for change.

Of course, election outcomes have proved to be the best single predictor of the direction of health policy reform in New Zealand. The 1996 election weakened the use of market-based mechanisms. Then, in late 1999, Labour was elected to office in coalition with the staunchly social democratic Alliance Party, and the new government pledged further health reform of a different stripe. The new Minister of Health Annette King introduced the New Zealand Public Health and Disability Bill into Parliament in August 2000. The Minister of Health reiterated her election promises that the government would establish:

> ... a New Zealand public health service that was based on co-operation and collaboration, that we were going to replace the current commercial and competitive model, that we were going to ensure that local communities once again had a say in the running of health services, and that we were going to focus on improving people's health as the fundamental role of a health service (*Evening Post*, 2000).

While several of the ideas outlined by the new Minister were already under implementation by the HFA, Labour's 1999 election promises required the creation of twenty-one new District Health Boards. DHBs would be responsible for health services in their areas, and act as both purchasers and providers. Transitional (non-elected) boards were established on 1 January 2001 and the first elections for the DHBs were held in October 2001. The legislation intended to 'provide a community voice' on decisions (New Zealand Public Health and Disability Act 2000, Section 1). DHBs have seven elected members and up to four appointed by the Minister of Health. Whereas the 1993 legislation had allowed the Ministers of Health and Finance to appoint 'whomever they thought would best achieve the objectives of the Crown Health Enterprise' (Health and Disability Services Act, 1993), the 2000 legislation requires the Minister of Health to appoint board members on the basis of both skills and representation, with a requirement that two members must be Māori. The emphasis on Māori representation reflected the coalition of Labour with the Alliance-affiliated Manu Motuhake Party, a party representing Māori.

The new legislation stringently codified the expectations for public oversight and participation, particularly consultation requirements, and thus gave the governance of local health services back to local communities, where it had been prior to the 1990s. The Act treated DHBs as if they were local authorities, which meant they had greater community consultation requirements than central government (see New Zealand Public Health and Disability Act 2000, Section 3, Subsection 38). The new Act required that board meetings be open to the public, and consultation on strategic planning. The 1993 reform legislation contained no requirements that CHEs consult the public, although purchasers (the RHAs and later the HFA) and the Core Services Committee, and then the National Health Committee, were required to consult the public (Health and Disability Services Act 1993 Section I, subsection 18).

Since the 2000 Act, the government is required to facilitate access to the health care system and to disseminate information about it (New Zealand Public Health and Disability Act 2000, Section 1). Previously, commercially oriented health care policies substantially weakened both public and parliamentary oversight and control of public hospitals. For example, hospitals frequently refused to release data to journalists and interest groups seeking information about the performance of the health care system. In 1995, when a newspaper requested information about hospital performance, data was actually supplied but with material relating to hospital safety deleted (Maling, 1995). And journalists' requests under official information legislation for statistics or financial data were frequently denied on the grounds that information of a commercial nature could be withheld from the public, in case other hospitals gained advantage in contracting with purchasers.

The Office of the Minister of Health has increased powers and responsibilities in the DHB system. The Minister of Health sets the overall policy direction for the health care system and has ministerial oversight responsibilities, and DHBs are required to follow. Under the prior internal market legislation, ministerial control was less defined but control over purchasers and providers increased as decision-making was increasingly centralised.

The Labour–Alliance reform package set in train yet another involved and costly process of change, with wide-ranging questions over whether the extent of change was justifiable. The processes of change and parallel policy developments have been detailed elsewhere (Gauld, 2009). The next chapter of this book looks at how well the DHB system, with its focus on community governance and elected representation, has performed.

CHAPTER **EIGHT**

The establishment and performance of District Health Boards

A S NOTED in the previous chapter, the District Health Board (DHB) system was the brain-child of the Labour-led Coalition Government, elected in 1999. In contrast to prior reforms of the New Zealand health system, the DHB reforms have remained relatively stable. In the period since their implementation, which occurred through the early part of the 2000s, after the New Zealand Public Health and Disability Act 2000 was passed, until the election of a National-led Coalition Government in 2008, there were only minor changes to the core structures for governing and funding the health system. The post-2008 government maintained the basic DHB structures. However, it subsequently sought to redesign various components of the system, while focusing on a different set of policy goals from the Labour-led governments.[1]

This chapter considers the establishment and performance of the DHB system, which remains the only example in the world of a publicly funded national health care system governed for an extended period by locally elected boards. With four sets of board elections including the inaugural ones in 2001, there is now considerable experience and research that can be drawn upon to inform discussion about governance of the DHB system and the performance of elected boards. Moreover, the system itself has been the subject of much scrutiny. This chapter reviews the process of creating DHBs, their structure, and other policy developments which have

---

1. Parts of this chapter draw upon discussions in Gauld (2009).

had implications for the performance of the DHB system, and it discusses the electoral component of the DHBs, considered by the Labour-led Government to be crucial for rejuvenating public involvement in health care governance and decision-making. In particular, we ask whether New Zealand's predominantly elected boards have achieved their goal of democratising governance and look at their capacity to preside over a high-performing health system. Finally, the chapter looks at reviews of the system by the National-led post-2008 government and the consequent changes. These highlight, and attempt to rectify, what are seen to be serious shortcomings in the DHB system and its governance arrangements. Notably, most of the changes made by the National-led government are occurring beyond the scope of the boards themselves, bringing into question their role in the system.

Creating the DHBs

As discussed in the previous chapter, the Labour-led Coalition Government sought a structure for the health care system that would engender public participation and involvement in governance, planning, and decision-making processes. It was in the spirit of this objective that the DHB structures were conceived. Two key DHB structures reflected that spirit: first, the creation of governing boards, with a majority of elected members and meetings open to the public; and second, the requirement for 'consultation' with the public and key stakeholder groups in all DHB work and decision-making.

The initial period following the 1999 general election saw the new DHB organisational structures put in place and the creation of a legislative framework for this structure. There was an intensive implementation programme, with committees and working groups within the Ministry of Health and the Health Funding Authority (in existence until late 2000, when it merged with the Ministry) focusing on developing different components of the new system, such as funding and accountability arrangements and how the principles of the Treaty of Waitangi would be represented in DHB structures. In keeping with the Labour-led Government's policy of transparency and openness, a series of Cabinet policy papers were made public. This shared information approach contrasted significantly with the health care reform of the mid-1980s and early 1990s.

Cabinet papers spelled out key decisions and rationales for the new elements of the DHBs – including the creation of elected boards. Notably, DHBs would each have eleven members, seven of whom would be elected by their local voting communities, and four of whom, including the chairperson and deputy, would be appointed by the Minister of Health. A DHB governing board would be responsible for the appointment and performance of the DHB chief executive, with the chief executive then responsible for the day-to-day performance of the entity itself. In a first for government policy, and enshrined in legislation, each DHB was to have at least two Māori members. They were also required to have a formal relationship with Māori tribes located within their regional boundaries.

Accountability arrangements, subsequently spelled out in the New Zealand Public Health and Disability Act 2000, were also the focus of considerable deliberation. DHBs are funded by central government via the Ministry of Health. They are accountable to the public through the Minister of Health and the government of the day. Thus, they are required to implement government policy and their activities and performance are a potential political risk. However, with elected membership, DHBs also have accountability to their electors and local communities. The enabling legislation dealt with this issue by stating that DHB members are accountable first and foremost to the minister and government. What DHBs were to be accountable for was to be expressed through the annual planning and five-yearly strategic planning process, with the content of annual plans subject to considerable review and oversight by the Ministry of Health. DHB funding would be contingent on a plan being agreed to by the Ministry. A section within the legislation lays out the various sanctions that the government could place on a DHB that fails to perform, with ramifications for the tension between central and local accountability. A DHB governing board that does not perform to the expectations of the Minister of Health can be subject to differing levels of central government monitoring or, at worst, dismissed and replaced by a commissioner. It is extremely difficult for a board and its elected members to challenge government policy or speak out about issues on behalf of their local communities that may pose risks for the Minister of Health. In sum, elected DHB members are in the rather unusual position of being local 'representatives' with little capacity to do much more than represent central government. In this sense, they differ markedly from other local bodies, such as city and district councils, and they differ significantly from the historically independent hospital boards.

The responsibility for creating DHBs was handed to the incumbent chief executive in each of the twenty-two existing hospital and health service regions (in place from 1997–2000). A merger of districts during this process meant twenty-one DHBs came into being. Each district was directed to work through a series of 'transition' phases, including drafting a plan for becoming a DHB and building a DHB infrastructure (including structures for ownership and management of public hospitals). The new DHBs also had to prove they had the capacity to assume the role of local services purchaser. Previously, purchasing had been the responsibility of the Health Funding Authority. Under the new legislation, purchasing was split between the Ministry of Health and the new DHBs. Before funds could be transferred from the Ministry of Health, DHBs would have to demonstrate that they had the capacity for local services purchasing. DHB creation also meant developing a governance structure in anticipation of the inaugural elections of 2001. Each of the twenty-one DHBs required support staff in areas such as finance, planning and services purchasing and a supporting infrastructure for this.

The expectations for DHBs were outlined in the *New Zealand Health Strategy* (King, 2000), which DHBs had to respond to in their annual and strategic plans and to which they would be held accountable. The report outlined a series of national goals and targets, such as improving access to elective services, developing primary care, reducing the incidence of diabetes, cancers and cardiovascular disease, reducing health inequalities and improving the health of the young and older people and those of Māori and Pacific ethnicity.

During the transitional phase, DHBs had to involve the public and key health sector stakeholders in planning and decision-making; each DHB-designate had to show 'how it intends to bring its community along with it' (Ministry of Health, 2000). Part of this process was (and continues to be) facilitated through the district 'needs assessment' that each DHB must conduct. The needs assessment involves assessing and modelling population health needs, and an appropriate mix of services to meet those needs. The needs assessment is one of the most important components of DHB activities and requires planning and prioritising within the fixed budgets that the DHBs are allocated by government.

DHBs went about the needs assessments in different ways. Some grouped together and used the services of an independent contractor to conduct needs assessments on their behalf. Others undertook their own assessments. The Hutt Valley DHB had possibly the most involved consultative process, which resulted in explicit lists of prioritised services and target populations for these services. However, to be fair, few questions were posed around the vast majority of services traditionally provided by the DHB (Hefford and De Boer, 2003). Rather, they occurred around the margins. Any public engagement around these services was limited and they still remain largely off the consultative agenda. The exception is where questions arise over service configuration, as discussed later in this chapter.

Creating the DHB boards: elections and democratisation

The DHBs and their governing boards were formally created under the New Zealand Public Health and Disability Act, which was passed at the end of 2000. The Labour-led Government had to include a number of amendments to garner the support of minor parties during the final readings of the legislation in Parliament. These changes included creation of central committees, such as the Public Health Advisory Committee, and mortality review committees. The legislation outlined the formal structures required of each DHB, including the governing board and its composition, as well as three sub-committees of the board: a public health committee to focus on how to improve population health, a hospital advisory committee to oversee the management of public hospitals, and a disability support services committee. These committees would be comprised of DHB board members and others from the local community appointed for their specific expertise or experience. Sub-committee meetings were also to be open to the public.

The governing boards themselves were not formally in place until after the inaugural DHB elections of late 2001. New Zealand has since had three DHB elections, in 2004, 2007 and 2010. The elections are held in conjunction with triennial local city council, regional council and community board elections. Local elections use the 'First Past the Post' electoral system, which was the method used for the inaugural 2001 DHB elections but adapted later (see below). In 2001, DHB regions (built around the pre-existing hospital regions for the reason that the Government did not wish to create additional disruption) were broken into wards to ensure representation across diverse geographic and demographic areas; typically, these were urban and rural and contained anything from one to five seats, depending on the size of the ward population. The DHB regions and wards did not correspond with local and regional government boundaries.

Local government officials were responsible for conducting DHB elections, including educating the public about DHB elections, receiving nominations, and facilitating polling. About a month before the election closing date, voting papers were mailed to all registered voters, along with other local government voting papers. Voting packs included booklets containing candidate photographs and profiles of up to around 200 words provided by the candidates themselves.

Central government also launched a public education drive to announce that candidate nominations were open and elections imminent. This included television, newspaper and movie theatre advertisements, creation of an election telephone info-line, and a household direct mail campaign. Government information consisted of overviews of the DHB system, highlighting the aim of public participation in health care governance. A particular note was made of the fact that the elections offered individuals the opportunity to participate as candidates and voters.

Arrangements for subsequent DHB elections were largely the same as in 2001, except that the Single Transferrable Vote system (STV) was mandatory; political leaders felt that it was a fairer system than First Past the Post. STV was optional for other local body polls, and most continued to use First Past the Post. Under STV voters rank candidates in order of preference. Candidates have to reach a certain quota of votes, which is based on the number of voters and candidates; once a candidate has reached that quota, additional votes for that candidate are discarded and 'surplus' votes shifted to voters' next ranked candidates, until the next most-preferred candidate reaches the quota (Farrell, 2001). The use of STV meant localised wards were abolished in favour of pan-DHB region electorates. The STV method was also used in Scotland's 2010 health board elections.

Candidates

As illustrated in Table 8, there was considerable candidate interest in the inaugural 2001 elections, which has diminished through subsequent elections. One thousand and eighty-four candidates contested 146 out of 147 seats (one seat had only one candidate), meaning there were 7.4 candidates per contested seat. Some wards attracted high candidate numbers. For instance, voters in the Waitakere ward, one of three composing the Waitemata DHB, had a choice of fifty candidates contending three seats. In the Christchurch ward, seventy-five candidates contested five seats. While it is difficult to know why some seats attracted so many candidates, it is possible that some were vying for what may have been seen as a lucrative post, with DHB membership paying around

Table 8. District Health Board candidate characteristics 2001–10

Seats and candidates	2001	2004	2007	2010
Seats contested	146	147	147	140
Total candidates	1084	518	428	371
Candidates per seat	7.4	3.5	2.9	2.6
Incumbent candidates as a percentage of contestable seats	7	24	28	32
Male (%)	55	57	58	59
Māori (%)	12	13	11	n/a
Voters				
Voter turnout (%)	50	42	43	49
Blank or invalid votes (%)	6	15	17	16

Source: collated by authors from data supplied by the Ministry of Health and Ministry of Internal Affairs.

$25,000 per year for about thirty days' service. Across the country, 55 per cent of candidates were male, 12 per cent were of Māori ethnicity, 7 per cent of candidates were incumbent board appointees and 5 per cent were DHB employees. Perhaps predictably, given the different objectives and potential for greater politicisation inherent within the DHB system, only around half of the pre-2001 appointed incumbents decided to stand for election.

In subsequent elections, the number of candidates has progressively fallen. Reasons for this remain unclear, but could correspond with the diffusion of knowledge about the contextual constraints on DHBs discussed below, as well as the presence of incumbents. The gender split in all three elections was roughly similar, as was the number of Māori candidates. There was a substantial increase from 2004 in the proportion of incumbent candidates (over 80 per cent of incumbents stood for election in both polls). In some DHB electorates there continued to be a large number of candidates. For example, the Capital Coast and Counties Manukau DHBs had forty and forty-one candidates respectively, and others had over thirty. However, the at-large electorates meant candidates were vying for seven seats.

Fifty per cent of voters voted in DHB elections in 2001. The turnout rate decreased in the following two elections but in 2010 it increased to 49 per cent (Table 8). After 2001, a significant number of voting papers were returned either blank or incorrectly filled out, rendering them invalid and reducing the overall proportion of votes that counted. Voters may have been confused by the STV voting system.

Election outcomes

The percentage of seats filled by incumbents in 2004 and 2007 increased, probably because the proportion of incumbent candidates standing was also higher. Candidates from a range of professions and backgrounds were elected in 2001. For instance, 37 per cent had experience in the 'health professions' including medicine, nursing and pharmacy, 31 per cent had worked in business or law or had company director/analysis experience, and at least 11 per cent had backgrounds in community work and advocacy. In 2004, 12 per cent of those elected were employed by the DHBs they were elected to. More than half had prior experience in local government. By 2007, over 70 per cent had such experience, but the proportion of DHB employees elected dropped to 6 per cent.

In many wards, more candidates stood for election in 2001 than in other years. As a result, most DHB members were elected with a small percentage of total votes. For example, in the Tauranga ward (33 candidates; three seats) 87,485 votes were received from 45 per cent of eligible voters, each of whom was able to vote for up to three candidates. The three successful candidates received 23,160 votes between them (26.47 per cent of the total). Comparing the 2004 and 2007 elections is difficult after the introduction of the STV voting system and at-large electorates, but the same pattern was observed: only a small proportion of voters backed each of the seven successful candidates in each DHB electorate.

The proportion of boards with Māori, Pacific or other minorities has increased since 2001. The advent of more appointed Māori board members has increased the total proportion of Māori board members. Along with the required Māori appointees, the government also added other Māori appointees with a range of skills pertinent to board governance. However, the percentage of Māori appointees on boards still remains below the proportion of Māori in the general population – 15 per cent. Moreover, few board members are from other minority groups.

Table 9. Characteristics of District Health Board members elected 2001–10

(%)	2001	2004	2007	2010
Incumbents as a % of all contestable seats	36	56	66	64
Māori	3	8	8	n/a
Gender: Male	56	58	54	54
Currently employed by the District Health Board	12	n/a	6	n/a

Source: collated by authors from data supplied by the Ministry of Health and Ministry of Internal Affairs.

Voter Behaviour

Voters faced a large number of choices in all three elections. In 2001, they had few incumbents to choose from, and most candidates lacked experience in DHB governance. To investigate voter behaviour, we conducted a fixed-response telephone survey of 500 voters, randomly selected from telephone directories, immediately following each election. In 2001, 100 respondents were sampled from each of five wards with large candidate numbers, representing rural and urban areas in the North and South Islands of New Zealand. In 2004 and 2007, five DHB electorates were targeted with a similar sampling approach (the survey was not conducted after the 2010 elections). The surveys had a margin of error of 4.3 per cent.

In both the 2001 and 2004 surveys, 65 per cent of respondents had voted in the DHB elections, suggesting the survey sample was not wholly representative of the general voting population. In 2007, 53 per cent had voted, which was closer to the election turnout, but still not representative. Non-voters were asked why they had not voted (Table 10). Notably, the number of voters who had not heard about the elections increased in 2004 and 2007. Also notable is the proportion of voters in all three elections who did not receive voting papers.

Respondents were asked how they made their choices from among the multiple candidates. The candidate profiles supplied with voting papers proved a useful information source for many. A proportion looked for candidates they knew. A small number resorted to guess work. Respondents were also asked about the main qualities they looked for in candidates. Responses for all three elections were similar, with a low

Table 10. Reasons non-voters gave for not voting in District Health Board elections, 2004–07

	2001	2004	2007
Respondents who said they did not vote	173	183	237
Didn't know about the elections	15	16	19
Didn't receive voting papers	12	18	12
No interest in elections	27	30	17
Don't know	20	28	35

Note: these categories are the highest scoring among a larger list of reasons that respondents could pick. Source: author survey.

Table 11. Factors influencing vote choice in District Health Board elections, 2004–07

(%)	2000	2004	2007
Voter used candidate profiles	61	53	64
Voter looked for someone they knew	26	35	27
Voter guessed	4	3	3
Experience in health service	57	61	56
Experience in community work	20	22	23
Experience in management/ financial matters	7	7	7

Note: these categories are the highest scoring among a larger list of reasons that respondents could pick. The numbers of people answering these questions were 327 (2001), 345 (2004), and 264 (2007). Source: author survey.

preference for candidates experienced in management and finance. Finally, in the 2004 and 2007 surveys, respondents were asked whether they found the STV system confusing and one third responded that it was confusing.

Appointed board members

Following the initial 2001 elections, the government released its list of DHB chairs and appointed members. Appointees were selected in accordance with a number of criteria, including the government's desire to ensure a complement of skills and experience around the board table. Over two thirds of appointees were incumbents and more than 60 per cent were Māori; the law requires each DHB to include two Māori members but not enough Māori were elected. A number of appointees had stood as candidates but failed to win seats. In 2004 and 2007, many sitting chairs were re-appointed to provide, as suggested by the Minister of Health, 'continuity and stability'. In 2010, around a third of chairpeople were replaced, sometimes controversially. Some who lost their positions said they were happy in their posts and had considerable support from health professionals and management. Several cross-board appointments were made to reflect the National-led Coalition Government's policy of regionalising planning and decision-making. Contrasting with 2001, there were few incumbents among appointees, but a similarly high percentage who self-identified as Māori.

Appointees hold an interesting position within DHBs. First, they are appointed by government, so there is potential for conflict between them and elected members. Research into this issue is very limited but there have been no reported cases of elected–appointed member clashes. If there were clashes, it is unlikely these would be aired in public as all DHBs have an agreement, rather like that of Cabinet, that they will speak publicly with one voice. Second, appointees' terms finish at election time, meaning they must wait to see if they are reappointed for another term. Third, it could be speculated that appointees may have potential for a better relationship with the government than elected members. Again, little is known about these dynamics.

How well have the DHBs performed?

The question of DHB performance is important, given the resources boards manage on behalf of the government and also the question of whether a predominantly elected board has the skill-mix to drive a strong performance. The answers are multifaceted and relate to both the governance arrangements, including the boards themselves, and the structure of the health care system.

A handful of formal evaluations of DHB performance have been conducted. One evaluation of the initial years of DHB development, released in 2007, suggested board members were relatively comfortable with the dual accountability to central government and local communities (Barnett et al., 2009, Barnett and Clayden, 2007).

The evaluations also found that central government goals and reporting frameworks were not supporting a population-based focus for local planning and service delivery (Mays et al., 2007), a problem encountered elsewhere in similar policy settings (Exworthy et al., 2002). In other words, DHBs were surrounded by conflicting objectives. Evidence from various sources suggests that DHBs and the post-2000 health system have experienced various problems.

First, as noted in the previous section, DHB elections and meetings have failed to engender strong public interest, although it could be argued – as politicians did early on – that the number of candidates standing for election represents a level of interest in local involvement in governance. While there are no hard data on it, the public has shown little interest in attending DHB meetings. Attendance tends to depend on the kinds of issues on the agenda. Meetings at which issues of high public interest are to be discussed attract more people. Often, according to journalists contacted when researching this book, the only attendees are local media. That said, DHB boards routinely conduct 'closed' sessions where potentially sensitive issues, such as finance, are discussed in private. Where DHBs have arranged special public meetings on particular issues on which they have sought public consultation, low turnout has also been a problem. However, there have been cases when DHB proposals to downsize or close services in remote areas have filled large halls with people. The requirement to consult with the public has been important, however. In some cases, following public feedback and deliberative processes, significant policy adjustments have been made. For example, in 2007, the Otago DHB, reflecting public input, withdrew a plan to institute charges for patients attending the emergency department with conditions amenable to treatment by a community-based general practitioner. This may not have happened under the prior system of corporate-style appointed boards that worked entirely away from the public gaze.

Second, it is not clear that the boards have been able to provide the all-important capacity expected of a governing board to drive innovation, monitor and question the performance of providers, and act as a sounding board for the chief executive and other full-time employees, because boards lack the expertise needed in several key areas. While data are limited, chief executives say that they often work in a vacuum; on the one hand having to educate the board about issues facing the DHB, while on the other making decisions that the board is not adequately equipped to discuss in any depth. The gaps in expertise range across a variety of areas, from finance and accounting to clinical governance, information technology, quality improvement and primary care. Effort in these areas can result in improved performance (Chaudry et al., 2006; Crump and Adil, 2009; Starfield et al., 2005). As further discussed below, primary care has suffered where boards have not had members with an appreciation for it, experience, or training in the field. For example, in a high profile and controversial case an Otago DHB board chairperson was dismissed because over a lengthy period their chief information officer had defrauded the board of $16 million through alleged information technology (IT) support purchases from companies he owned that delivered no service to the board. Had the board had the expertise to scrutinise information technology purchases and activities more knowledgeably, the fraud may not have been possible.

The gap in skills and expertise is particularly acute in the area of information technology, which is recognised worldwide as a driver of system improvement and integration. Likewise, quality improvement has been on the international health policy agenda for several years, with studies demonstrating that health care organisations that invest in quality have reduced costs, a happier workforce, and better health outcomes. Yet most boards have failed to embrace IT or quality improvement. The situation has been the same with clinical governance, where (as noted in Chapter One) the idea that clinically led and team-based work, and partnerships between management and clinicians in the running of hospitals and health care organisations, produce more efficient and higher quality health care delivery. Until government began initiatives in this area, discussed below, boards have paid only limited attention to clinical governance.

Third, and to be fair, most DHBs have been focused on austerity and the 'bottom line'. As noted, they must live within annual central government budget allocations as determined by a Population-based Funding Formula (PBF). This provides a dollar amount per person per region, weighted for various characteristics, including ethnicity, socio-economic status as measured by the New Zealand Index of Deprivation, and the composition of rural and urban population. For example, the South Canterbury DHB serves a population that is considered 100 per cent rural, including the population of Timaru. The area has an older population, so the DHB receives considerably more payments per person than other DHBs. Age, and factors such as 'unmet need' in the community, also influence the level of funding. The PBF has evolved over the years, with periodic reviews and adjustments, such as increases to nurses' pay of around 20 per cent in the mid-2000s. However, the PBF serves some regions better than others. Those in the south, where populations are static and there are fewer Māori or people in the lower socio-economic groups, receive considerably less per capita than other DHBs. The southern areas have also been historically over-funded compared with DHBs in the north. Therefore the decline in funding for these DHBs has led to perpetual deficits, or funding levels that have not met with service demand. As a result, many DHBs have focused on reducing deficit levels. Board meetings and activities centre on how to reconfigure services so that expenditure can be kept in check, and preferably reduced.

The Capital Coast and the Otago (now part of the Southern DHB) DHBs are illustrative of the difficulties posed by the PBF and incapacity to generate income from other sources; all hospital services must be free of charge and access has few formal restrictions. In 2007, the Capital Coast Chief Executive resigned and the board was replaced by a commissioner, partly due to financial performance but also because of a series of quality lapses (Health and Disability Commissioner, 2007). In 2010, the chief executive that followed also resigned, as he saw no further room for cost cutting and was subject to ongoing pressure to bring the deficit level down. DHBs are periodically subject to different levels of financial monitoring by central government. This has proven controversial, as in the early 2000s for the Otago DHB. Neither the Ministry of Health nor the Otago DHB could agree on a plan for deficit reduction, with each suggesting the other's expectations were unacceptable. After a lengthy standoff, an independent assessor acted as a negotiator between the two parties, resulting in an eventual funding increase and an agreed plan for the way forward.

Various reports have implied that hospital efficiency has declined since the DHBs were created. Treasury, for instance, suggested efficiency had dropped by 2.6 per cent per annum in the first half of the 2000s, but increased by 1.1 per cent in the three years prior when the HFA was in place (Treasury, 2005). The Ministry of Health's 2008 briefing to the incoming government gave little reason to believe DHB efficiency had improved. It recommended better integration and planning of services, especially across the 'four regions' that replicate those of the former RHAs of the 1990s (Ministry of Health, 2008b). Of course, one explanation for the efficiency decrease is the doubling in health funding through the 2000s under the Labour-led Coalition Government, especially as the economy went through a period of considerable growth in the years before the global financial crisis of 2008. Much of this funding went into salary increases, more staff, new facilities and primary care reforms. Another is the often-cited one – mirroring historical discussions around the number of hospital boards – that twenty-one DHBs were simply too many, working against economies of scale, requiring considerable duplication of functions across twenty-one administrative and service delivery systems, and countering national planning, coordination and knowledge transfer. That said, the question of efficiency throughout the DHB period remains a point of conjecture, with emerging data implying that there may have been some improvements since 2007 (Desai, 2012).

Complicating the situation for both central government and DHBs, about a quarter of the services and funding that should have been purchased at the DHB level remained within the Ministry of Health, including maternity services, some mental health services, and primary care funding, among others. This meant that affected providers contracted with DHBs, but were paid by the Ministry, resulting in a convoluted and confusing set of administrative and funding arrangements, with high transaction costs.

However, between 2001 and 2008, population health indicators and DHB performance targets showed some improvement. Among ten specific service targets introduced in 2007 (which included increasing immunisation rates, reducing cancer waiting times, improving diabetes services) there were promising gains (Ministry of Health, 2008c). Health outcomes for New Zealanders, as measured by life expectancy, infant and cardiovascular mortality rates, showed advances in the 2000s. The health sector could claim some responsibility for this, although other factors such as improvements in the economy may also have contributed. Inequalities in health between Māori and other New Zealanders diminished. Smoking rates dropped and levels of obesity appeared to be stabilising (Ministry of Health, 2008b; Blakely et al., 2007), although New Zealand continued to have the third most obese population amongst OECD countries (OECD, 2009). That said, data show that several DHBs under-performed across various indicators. These included the extent to which they involved Māori in planning processes; produced strategies to improve service effectiveness; managed cardiovascular risk factors and put stroke services in place; developed quality and safety improvement systems; and facilitated patient enrolment in Care Plus primary health care programmes (Ministry of Health, 2008a). Performance in elective procedures – an area of considerable government and DHB policy activity – was mixed. There were significant differences in waiting times and access to comparable treatments across DHBs, and problems of consistency in how patients were prioritised. Of course, this indicates that while there may be systematic problems with the performance of the DHB system, there are also considerable differences by individual DHB. Contributing factors include the individual management systems, funding levels (as dictated by the funding formula discussed above) and service organisation.

One factor that complicated the DHB landscape and the work of the DHB boards was the establishment (from 2003) of Primary Health Organisations (PHOs), born out of the government's *Primary Health Care Strategy* (King, 2001). The DHBs must plan for and fund primary care services in their regions, so PHO creation became a DHB responsibility. Implementation of this has been discussed in some detail elsewhere (Gauld, 2008). The Labour-led Government's goals of reducing patient fees, improving access, improving services for those with chronic disease, formally enrolling patients with a primary care provider, and building multi-disciplinary team-based approaches to primary care delivery were laudable. However, the Government made a poor job of implementation by failing to provide clear and ongoing oversight and direction to the sector. This complicated the situation for both PHOs and DHBs, who had to work out many of the details of what PHOs should look like and what sorts of programmes they should develop. Government gave PHOs an additional $500 million per year (a 6–7 per cent increase in health expenditure) over six years, beginning in 2002. With an implicit anti private practice stance, the Government failed to seek to partner with general practitioners to build PHOs (Gauld, 2008). This led to a crucial lack of support from GPs. The result was that the Government allowed any organisation that fulfilled its basic requirements to become a PHO.

By 2005, there were around eighty PHOs, ranging in size from a few thousand to over 350,000 enrolled patients. A multitude of problems emerged, including a lack of managerial capacity in many smaller PHOs that needed the services of GP-backed independent practitioner associations with ready-made infrastructure for patient data collection, enrolment, chronic disease management programmes, and so on. Some DHBs were more supportive of PHOs than others, as reflected in availability of funding and other backing for PHO initiatives. PHO leaders note many board members lacked a good understanding of the benefits of effective primary care, which made it difficult to gain support and funding from DHBs for new initiatives. DHB management did not include sufficient primary-care expertise in the planning and funding team (Gauld, 2008).

The failure to articulate a vision regarding primary care development was a crucial lost opportunity both for central government and the DHBs. This was due partly to a failure to think through the implications of parallel DHB and PHO planning structures. PHOs, arriving a couple of years after DHBs, seemed to be an add-on. Issues such as how best to configure a PHO, or to integrate services within or between regions, had not been worked through. The funding model for PHOs was an obstacle to bringing the range of primary care practitioners together within a single organisation. Pharmacists, midwives and other allied care providers remained separately funded: there was no financial incentive stimulating all primary care providers within a region to work together in a PHO. But, there was also a failure by the Ministry of Health to outline the level at which primary care fees should ultimately be set, or whether the goal was to minimise co-payments. Ongoing uncertainty also surrounded such questions as whether PHOs should work to manage extended budgets for hospital and other services on behalf of patients, whether they should compete with one another or be territorial monopolies, and whether all primary care work, including district health nursing administered by Public Health Services, should be integrated within PHOs.

The post-2008 approach

The 2008 general election saw the formation of a new National-led Coalition Government. The new Government pledged that it would not make any structural changes to the health system during its term, and so it was committed to the DHBs. However, as noted above, by the latter part of the 2000s, serious questions about the performance of the health system had begun to emerge. The arrival of the new Government also coincided with the global financial crisis, creating a less than favourable environment for public service expenditure. Two sets of issues confronted the Government. First, the structures for planning, funding and delivering health services had become increasingly complex, with widespread recognition that the duplication in administrative systems across the DHBs added little value and limited the capacity to coordinate the system centrally or improve its performance. Second, the financial crisis meant the government needed to consider options for curbing health expenditure increases, or working more effectively within available funding.

The Government took various steps to tackle these issues, in a policy agenda that has parallels with developments in the English NHS (Whitehead et al., 2010). Key policy directions include the introduction of six health sector targets, including reduced waiting times in hospital emergency departments, improved access to elective surgery, increased immunisation levels, improved cancer, diabetes and cardiovascular services, and better help to quit for smokers. From 2010, the targets have been published quarterly by the Ministry of Health, showing how DHB performances compare against benchmarks. They have become a core focus for DHBs and their boards as they seek to meet benchmark standards.

For many DHBs, satisfying the emergency department target that 95 per cent of patients will be admitted, discharged or transferred within six hours has been a challenge. This is desirable as the Minister of Health sees it as an indicator of broader hospital performance: studies show long delays in the emergency department suggest inadequate attention is being paid to the way in which patients flow through the hospital (Ben Tovim et al., 2008). Simple remedies, such as doctors conducting ward rounds earlier in the day, can free up beds and in turn allow patients to be transferred from the emergency department and admitted to hospital as in-patients. Boards have concentrated their efforts on the re-design of internal hospital organisational systems, involving clinicians in this process. This has propelled an emphasis on 'clinical governance' and 'clinical leadership', a central theme of the report of a Ministerial Review Group (MRG) to the Minister of Health in 2009.

The Minister established the MRG shortly after the National-led Government assumed office in late 2008 and was chaired by a former Treasury chief, Murray Horn. The MRG was asked to report on how to improve the performance of health sector, in particular how to curtail expenditure, reduce duplication and improve quality. The MRG report reiterated the shortcomings with the DHB system outlined earlier in this chapter and provided a series of recommendations for change (Ministerial Review Group, 2009). Most of these have subsequently become government policy. The recommendations were:

- Streamline 'back office' systems, including finance, planning, human resources, health information technology, procurement and other functions as appropriate.
- Increase the emphasis on quality improvement, including the creation of a separate national agency.

- Establish a mechanism for health technology assessment (comparative effectiveness research).
- Reduce the number of DHBs and PHOs, or at least the duplication across multiple parallel organisations.
- Regionalise DHB planning to ensure inter-regional equity and reduce administration.
- Improve system productivity, especially the provision of timely access to and availability of care.

To operationalise the recommendations, a new National Health Board (NHB) was created in 2009. The NHB was established in the Ministry of Health for political reasons: the National Party had pledged there would be no 'major health sector restructuring'. A separate agency would have made the government vulnerable to the allegation of breaking that promise. That said, the NHB effectively operates independently, with its own governing board and chief executive. The NHB initially inherited more than half the Ministry's staff, but is expected to reduce the number of staff over time. Its primary aim is to improve DHB performance and, in conjunction with the new Health Benefits Limited, to centralise various back office functions in an effort to reduce duplication, costs, and administrative staff at the DHB level. Other roles include working out which services should remain centrally planned and funded and which should be the responsibility of DHBs. The NHB also houses the National Health IT Board (aiming at national consistency in IT standards and fully portable electronic patient records by 2014), Health Workforce New Zealand (which works on workforce development issues), and the Capital Development Committee (aimed at bringing consistency to the processes for capital development funding allocation). Thus, many of the issues and decisions that fell within the realm of individual DHBs and their boards are gradually being removed from the local level.

The NHB is also seeking improvements in areas such as clinical governance and is asking DHBs to identify and support clinical leaders in developing management–clinician partnerships for decision-making, and to report back to the NHB on progress made. Boards also have to renew inter-regional planning efforts towards reducing duplication and focusing on a broader shared population base. For example, some DHBs – such as those in the central North Island – are working on creating clinical networks for in-demand services where specialists such as pediatric oncologists and neurosurgeons may be in short supply. The Ministry itself is focusing on the more traditional role of sector monitoring and ministerial policy advice.

In addition to the NHB, in late 2010 the Government created an independent Health Quality and Safety Commission intended to promote quality improvement, as well as continue the work of the former Quality Improvement Committee. This included producing an annual 'sentinel event' report (Quality Improvement Committee, 2009). The Quality Commission is expected to work with DHBs on governance and process issues aimed at improving patient safety and reducing medical errors. Studies suggest medical errors affect around 12 per cent of patients in New Zealand and could account for up to 30 per cent of health expenditure (Davis et al., 2002; Health Committee, 2006).

The NHB recommended national investment in health technology assessment and comparative effectiveness analysis. This would mean that services would be funded according to the evidence as to their effectiveness. At the time of writing, the National Health Committee was undergoing a reconfiguration to focus on effectiveness questions. Pharmac, the government's independent drug-buying agency that has expertise in technology assessment techniques, had also agreed to assess a limited number of medical devices.

The Minister of Health has sought a reduction in the number of PHOs in order to reduce the level of expenditure on back office administration and eradicate many of the smaller PHOs, instructing DHBs to preside over this. At the time of writing, a series of mergers between smaller PHOs have produced around thirty in operation. In keeping with the National Party's pre-election policy statement, *Better, Sooner, More Convenient*, the Government has commissioned the establishment of nine Integrated Family Health Centre pilots, in the hope that more than 70 per cent of New Zealanders will be enrolled with such a centre by around 2013. These centres are intended to offer around-the-clock primary care services, feature a multi-disciplinary practitioner base, and have extended diagnostic and (some) specialist services. Gazing into the crystal ball, and harking back to developments led by Independent Practitioner Associations in the late 1990s (Malcolm et al., 1999), it is possible that stronger centres will increasingly take on DHB planning and purchasing functions for their populations, coordinating and offering services provided by a network of providers including public hospitals, from a primary care base. The expansion of PHOs could potentially reduce the relevance of DHBs or undermine their role, especially if the NHB funds PHOs directly.

Finally, the Minister of Health has noted concerns about the capacity of DHB boards to govern effectively, and particularly about whether members have the required skills to drive performance improvement, especially financial performance (Birchfield and Mueller, 2010). As noted, DHB members now receive post-election training from the Ministry of Health. This has tended to be focused on the role of board members in the health system and the legislative framework within which they must work, with limited focus on performance-related issues. The Minister has suggested additional training and mentoring may be required.

Conclusion

This chapter has reviewed an important period in the history of New Zealand's health system, which was significant for two reasons. First, following the era of corporate governance through the 1990s, the period represents the reassertion of the democratic governance model and the localisation of decision-making through the creation of DHBs. Second, it provides information on the operation of a health system that is democratically governed.

The policies that led to the DHB system being created were a result of political party politics, particularly the ideas of the Labour Party. In several respects, they were a response to those of the prior decade of National Party leadership and were produced despite that fact that from the late 1990s there had been considerable movement away from National's notions of competition. While Labour's prescription provided a solid foundation in line with international thinking about how to improve health systems and health status – with its focus on public participation, primary care, reducing inequalities, and population-based goals and targets – the institutional design and execution of the prescription was quite possibly its undoing. The key structures, twenty-one DHBs and multiple PHOs, proved to be administratively unwieldy; by the end of Labour's reign, its prescription appeared to be faltering. The public had not rushed to the polls to elect DHB representatives, while the representatives themselves seemed to have limited capacity to do much at all beyond implement central government policy. Indeed, there were even questions about the capacity of elected members to provide the skills and experience required for sound health system governance.

The change in government at the 2008 general elections provided a new National-led Coalition Government with the impetus to once again review the governance and organisation of the health system. Following the Ministerial Review Group's recommendations, and with pledges not to 'restructure', the Government retained the core DHB structures. However, in tandem, it has created a series of new agencies designed to exact improved health system performances in key policy areas while, in an evolutionary manner, reducing local decision-making capacity through centralising various administrative functions. This signifies an emerging model aimed at national consistency and oversight that includes local input into local health service governance, while gradually requiring that DHBs and other providers comply with centrally determined policy and performance standards. In the next and final chapter we look at key lessons from the experiences with democratic health care governance in New Zealand and consider alternatives.

CHAPTER NINE

Conclusion: realism and representation

THERE ARE FIVE lessons to be drawn from this analysis of elected representation. First, apart from a brief interlude in the 1990s, elected boards seem to have been resilient to change at least partly because of their nineteenth-century origins; hospital boards established a position of strength before national health insurance was created, as discussed in Chapter Three. As most people are not familiar with the story of New Zealand hospitals or how health boards started, we traced the origins of the hospitals and their changing relationship with and gradual financial dependence on central government. Hospital boards outlived the many challenges to their existence. We have described how the hospital benefit was created without changing the organisation of health services, as happened in many other countries.

The second lesson is about board and community recalcitrance, and their fear of losing control of their hospitals. Boards leveraged power to repeatedly make hospital reform an election issue, with support from other stakeholders. Boards had community and electoral support at the periphery and that support extended nationally through general elections. The politics at the local level were not contained, but looped in a feedback process to national politics.

A third lesson is that political elites and the public sometimes used elected boards strategically to advance values and ideologies. Boards have represented differing prevailing ideals in society. Ultimately, New Zealanders could benefit from distinguishing between the symbolic ideals of elected health boards and the actual task of operating a billion-dollar enterprise. Boards have taken on roles for which they were not necessarily designed. At times the model of elected boards has been a poster-child for democracy and at other times a contrast to market choice. By taking a *realist* approach to the meaning of health boards, we can ask whether we have conflated local control with local community survival and as a result set ourselves up for failure by confusing the only alternatives as unresponsive, bureaucratically administered, or market-oriented health services.

The fourth lesson drawn from analysing some of the purposes of elected boards through history is the need for more conceptual clarity around the goals and meaning of elected representation in the health service. Without the insights gained from an historical perspective there can be a failure to grasp fully the purposes and benefits of elected representatives. When people decide to prioritise representation and geography as the most important value in health governance arrangements, there are going to be tradeoffs, and the related fifth lesson is that there is a price to pay for defining our health system along geographic lines, which may be health care 'system-ness' (see page 170). As we close this discussion, our final questions concern the future: is the health care system best served by elected local boards, and should we continue to have a democratic model of such boards?

Lesson 1: the evolution of hospital boards

The origins of hospital board power can be traced back to the early days of European settlement in the nineteenth century, when there were scattered and isolated communities, especially in the South Island. When New Zealand embarked on a national health programme, the historical strength of local government served to reinforce this power. The pattern of settlement initially produced a provincial constitutional structure, and early legislation gave hospital boards authority and encouraged localised forms of governance. Thus community control over hospitals was established as the norm.

The first six European settlements were isolated and independent: all traded independently with Great Britain. In some cases, local mail sent to addresses within New Zealand travelled via Sydney due to the better communication links with Australia (Morrell, 1964 [1932], p.22–25). Settlers saw themselves as belonging to separate local areas, not a nation, and they supported self-governance and freedom from control by London (see Morrell, 1964 [1932], Sutch, 1956). However, politicians in Great Britain did not support such radical federalism. Instead, they created a provincial system of government for New Zealand (Morrell, 1964 [1932]). From 1854 to 1876, New Zealand was divided into six provinces, which later became nine. Provincial governments governed provinces under the oversight of a national assembly but were abolished for a number of reasons, which included improved communications, limited finances, financial disparities between southern and northern colonies, and the development requirements of the nation, as well as the competitive feasible alternative of local government (Bush, 1980; Morrell, 1964 [1932]). (Provincial governments competed with local governments for funds and responsibilities.) Central government's growing need for uniformity in matters such as immigration also contributed (Morrell, 1964 [1932]). Once provincial governments were abolished, local governments assumed many of their functions and increased their own power (Bush, 1980). Local government expanded between 1875–76, with the number of counties increasing from thirty-nine to sixty-three. Further counties could be established if voter support exceeded 60 per cent (Bush, 1980). The subdivision of local administration was carried to extreme lengths, with hundreds of 'petty' local bodies providing stumbling blocks to the merging of local government units (Pember Reeves, [1898] 1950).

Who controlled hospitals after the demise of provincial government is disputed. Pember Reeves suggests that the control of hospitals was left to their boards (Pember Reeves, [1898] 1950). The Department of Health has claimed that, once the provincial governments were abolished, central government gained control of the hospitals (Department of Health, 1975, p.9), while Bush argues that counties and boroughs, acting as boards of health, controlled hospitals (Bush, 1980). Local boroughs seem to have retained control, since they managed to prevent government from reducing the number of hospitals (Oliver, 1977). Regardless of who eventually had control, early hospital board legislation (1885) gave hospital boards authority and encouraged localised forms of governance. These laws reinforced the idea of community control over hospitals.

Lesson 2: the recalcitrant power of hospital boards

The power of hospital boards ultimately depended on public support. Often overlooked, public preferences on health care shape policy development just as much as those of professionals and governments. In the United Kingdom and the United States, the development of the NHS and Medicare Acts were shaped by fundamental expectations of health care based on the different 'established understandings' in these countries (Jacobs, 1993). Health care institutions not only respond to, but can also *shape* public opinion. Public understandings are shaped by the organisation of health care, and these understandings feed back into policy. In New Zealand, the match between ideas and core political values may explain the longevity of hospital boards and their seeming monopoly in hospital policy. After establishing a degree of independence in the nineteenth century, boards drew strength in the twentieth century from two powerful supporting ideas that made their reform difficult: their relationships to hospitals, and their role in democratic representation.

Boards were well supported and connected to local communities and voters. People were more emotionally attached to hospitals than to boards. However, the linkage of hospitals to hospital boards let the latter survive parasitically on public support for the former. Hospitals had been established by local communities and in many smaller communities they continued to be a focus of civic pride. Reform or regionalism did not always want to change the hospitals, just the boards, but in many places, boards and hospitals were one and the same, and an attack on one was an attack on the other. Especially during the economic revolution of the 1980s, when rural and small-town New Zealand was undergoing economic dislocation, hospital boards drew power from the idea of local hospitals as the core of otherwise fragile communities. They were often seen as the special guardians of the hospitals in the communities in which they were located. Governments wanted to consolidate services regionally, but the core political value of 'ownership' of hospitals, along with the close ties between hospitals and their communities, made this policy difficult to enforce.

Reformers were not blind to these values, but found it difficult to challenge them, especially publicly. In every episode of reform, government officials either started the reform process with this knowledge or later became aware of the ties between hospital boards and communities. In 1953, John Marshall scrawled an imperative 'cannot close hospitals', and thirty years later, in 1987, consultants travelled throughout the country and found 'a deeply ingrown belief' that local health services (general practitioner and hospital facilities) within 20–30 kilometres are 'an inalienable right of New Zealanders ... Hospitals are part of the fabric of what New Zealanders regard as facilities that comprise a community. Threats of closure are met with considerable community concern' (National Archives, 1987).

Ambitious reformers in the 1980s wanted to cut the umbilical cord between hospitals and their boards and remove democratically elected representatives from those boards. This was a double whammy of community virtues under attack, and acutely felt in a time when hospital reform was one of many volleys from Wellington. As one Taskforce member said, 'Each citizen as a voter likes to feel he or she has some influence in governing the health services' (National Archives, 1988). These values endured even after elected boards were eradicated in the 1990s. A review of the sector in 1997 stressed the importance of participation and local communities' roles in health policy: 'Communities have the right to participate, and funders and providers are responsible for ensuring communities' values and preferences are reflected in decision-making' (Steering Group on the Implementation of the Coalition Agreement, 1997).

In actuality, the ideal of democracy in the health service was slightly different from the actual involvement of most citizens in hospital politics. Hospital boards did not always *represent* citizens explicitly, but the appearance of democracy was important within communities (National Archives, 1987). The low turnout in hospital board elections suggested that communities were not attached to them. As tools of actual democracy, they were probably less than adequate – democratic in formal structure but undemocratic in actual practice (Mulgan, 1984).

Voters were unlikely to be interested in the *details* of hospital governance, but hospital boards had a strong interest in revealing citizens' stakes in any policy reform directed towards hospitals or boards. Boards were able to rally voters around the possibility of hospital closures. Hospital board members were not shy about blaming local problems on national policies either, which meant that successive Ministers of Health faced the wrath and embarrassment of outspoken board members when they upset hospital boards. Criticism of ministers influenced the fortune of the governing party and all its members, so this was a powerful way of retaining the policies that boards favoured. Opposition members could also win support within local districts by promising to fight government policies that threatened local hospital boards.

The endurance of hospital boards suggests they embodied community values, whether or not people actually participated in local hospital politics. Hospital boards retained the support of their communities despite low participation, and when specific hospitals or hospital boards were under threat communities rallied in support of them. In short, hospital boards were not just 'organisations' that were 'lean, no nonsense' efficient tools for coordinating activities (Barnard, 1938). The boards were institutions, and institutions have deep roots in social needs and respond to those pressures as 'a responsive adaptive organism' (Selznick, 1957). An organisation becomes an institution once it is infused with value and symbolises community aspirations and sense of identity (Selznick, 1957). Expendability is a good test of institutionalisation: 'If an organisation is merely an instrument, it will be readily altered or cast aside when a more efficient tool becomes expendable. Most organisations are thus expendable' (Selznick, 1957). Reforms in the 1990s particularly sought to encourage this ethos of expendability through market mechanisms.

Lesson 3: the varying purposes of elected boards

That boards have served a variety of purposes has been overlooked in much scholarship on New Zealand health policy and policy-making. First, there is the strategic use of hospital boards, usually in moments of crisis. Some of the most consistent defenders have been national political elites who might (if they were in Cabinet) support reform at another time. While economic issues are usually at the core of voters' decisions at election time, hospital reform was prominent in elections in the 1970s and the 1990s. The electoral effects of hospital boards were never direct but still palpable for New Zealand politicians: the boards' power was latent, but anticipated as a potential threat. Theories of how politics work suggest that elected representatives are concerned about how the electorate will react to their record of performance, and it is the anticipated reaction of the electorate that motivates politicians (Arnold, 1990). Elected representatives have strong incentives to make the right inferences about public opinion, otherwise they will lose office to those who do so (Ferejohn, 1990). Although hospital reform was not enough to solely determine an election, it would bring embarrassment or negative attention to governments who attempted it. Hospital boards and their members lacked the formal powers of doctors to strike or not co-operate with government policies. But they were a crucial political ally or foe that governments had to consider in any reform proposal, giving them considerable political power, as the case studies demonstrate in the preceding chapters.

Political parties at the centre have piggy-backed on hospital reform. A more unkind characterisation is that they were often Janus-faced.

Sometimes Opposition parties used hospital reform to shore up their own support, and then proceeded to introduce similar policies. In some cases, such as in the 1980s, the potential liability of the Gibbs Taskforce was turned into an opportunity for credit-claiming: Labour won political points for rejecting the plans and proposing a more moderate version. Thus, boards have been used as vehicles for the promotion of political goals that are not necessarily those that will best benefit the public and patients.

A second political purpose saw boards used as pawns of larger schisms. Communities used the issue of proposed hospital reform to take a last stand against marketisation of New Zealand in the 1980s (Chapter Five) as the bulwark of defence against more privatisation. They were a focal point for voter discomfort with economic reforms that were initially hardest on the rural sector. Boards also provided a territory for political elites fighting larger ideological battles, not always along partisan lines (Labour maintained both ideologies simultaneously in the 1980s).[1] On the left, boards were said to provide representation and equity, and a foil against the business model. On the right, there was a distrust of representation and political 'meddling' by boards, underlaid by theories of agency capture that dovetailed with a low expectation of the efficiency of government. In the 1980s, the efficiency and managerial capacity of boards were a focus. Behind-the-scenes records revealed two views: either boards embodied community or they were bemoaned as organisations crying out for the discipline of the market. This split was also a reflection of differences between different agencies in Wellington that claimed jurisdiction over health policy – Treasury versus the Health Department/Ministry during the 1980s and 1990s.

The problem with these two alternatives is that they are polarised models of health care that offer limited visions: a case of either democracy or the market. Advocates of a market approach in the early 1990s said they would take politics (elected boards) out of decisions on health care and replace political decisions with market processes. But in order to engage in reform in 1991, Cabinet had to wrest control from local communities and concentrate power in the capital city, Wellington, and then redistribute

---

1. These battles originate in, and reflect, changing demographics and the rise of a transformed Labour Party in the 1970s: the same fissure that ultimately placed Finance Minister Roger Douglas supporters against Prime Minister David Lange in the late 1980s. What the right and left within Labour both agreed on was that boards did not do enough to support preventive care (thus winning the endorsement of public health supporters and activists) and boards did not reflect the needs of Māori.

it to regional purchasers. In 1999 and 2000, these ideas were turned on their head when Labour re-introduced elected boards. When the Minister of Health Annette King introduced the New Zealand Public Health and Disability Bill into Parliament in August 2000, she said Labour had made an election promise to create:

> ... a New Zealand public health service that was based on co-operation and collaboration, that we were going to replace the current commercial and competitive model, that we were going to ensure that local communities once again had a say in the running of health services, and that we were going to focus on improving people's health as the fundamental role of a health service (*Evening Post*, 2000).

The symbolic power of these statements is consistent with the speech by the Minister of Health in 1926 (see beginning of Chapter One) but both serve to illustrate how elected boards frequently become the battleground for larger debates about the role of the state, rather than simply the design of the health service. These values do serve to clarify deeply held views about the role of government in health care. But juxtaposed against the bold new market models promising an idealised market of health insurance choices proposed in the 1990s, the democratic ideal looks equally unable to address the nature of complex and geographically spread health care services. Neither of the ideals – market or democracy – provides an actual roadmap for developing high quality and accessible services.

The limitations of ideologically driven models are apparent when we consider the United States, where most private hospital boards (most are not-for-profit) are self-appointing. A key lesson from the US is that the best quality and most well-run hospitals are led by boards with strong clinical membership. This seems to translate, through a coherent clinical and management-focused strategy, into strong clinical leadership at the executive level of the organisation, with a focus on highly organised clinical systems and processes. This, in turn, translates into better quality of care and patient outcomes and, ultimately, reduced costs (Dorgan et al., 2010; Goodall, 2011; James and Savitz, 2011).

Lesson 4: representation has never been defined

Elected boards are promoted as vehicles for good governance and public involvement. The reality, however, has been far from the ideal. Chapters One and Eight noted the low civic involvement in electoral processes and board meetings, which questions the very legitimacy of their representative role. This has been particularly so in the contemporary DHB era, with voter turnouts rarely reaching 50 per cent and being further undermined by blank and invalid votes. In addition, the limited studies of DHB voter behaviour suggest that few make an informed candidate choice. Two factors may explain low turnout. First, when the expectations of the model are unclear the public may feel ambivalent about the purpose of elected boards. Proponents may offer few justifications for something they perceive as intrinsically good. Who can disagree with the idea of democracy? Second, the confusion can stem from the different assumptions about the nature of representation that also makes it hard to evaluate success. The meaning of representation is multi-faceted (Pitkin, 1972). Some discussions around elected boards and participation in general have implied a delegate model of representation. At other times, elected boards convey a direct democracy model of representation, where people's views on particular issues are heard in the process of policy development and decision-making. As discussed in Chapter Eight, we have limited knowledge of whether a delegate process occurs (anecdote suggests it may only be around specific issues), and we do not know whether that process changes policies. People could want different things from their representatives; some may want board members to be more like trustees – good stewards of the health service. The public might be more concerned about whether boards are providing high quality and accessible health care services. The lack of interest shown by the public may also reflect a lack of confidence that elected boards have the skills necessary to govern complex local health systems. As shown in Chapter Eight, data on the DHBs, now in place for over a decade, suggest that performance has been mediocre.

The murkiness around representation is driven by a third assumption: that it improves accountability. It may do so, but not always in the way people expect, which may prove disappointing. In theory, when change is needed the public may be more likely to accept a policy if they have an elected rather than an appointed representative or official. More cynically characterised, the purpose of retaining representation is to make unpopular decisions easier. Elected boards have rarely served to depoliticise the decision-making process or increase the acceptance of policies. Attempts to shift the blame to the local level sometimes boomerang back to the centre, since voters often (rightly or wrongly) perceive that unpopular decisions are actually being driven by central government.

Lesson 5: Tradeoffs between representation and 'system-ness'

The DHB system was created to restore local input to decision-making, but may have exacerbated the historical localism that characterises health care governance, administration and service delivery in New Zealand. DHBs have not worked collaboratively to develop and plan services, and localised control has worked against the development of a health care 'system', and instead facilitated the creation of multiple parallel local systems with their own executive management teams, budgets and planning processes, and configurations for service delivery. This lack of collaboration prompted legislation in 2010 to force more national and regional cooperation. Building consistent and integrated services is the focus of the world's leading health care systems, which have populations far larger than New Zealand's 4.5 million.

Similarly, although hospital deficits are a problem worldwide, many DHBs have failed to manage effectively within budget. One reason is that central government funding is allocated to the boards on a weighted population basis. Boards with higher proportions of older, lower socio-economic status, Māori or Pacific people receive additional funding, meaning some DHBs are in a better financial position than others because of the characteristics of the populations they serve. Recent investigations suggest operating deficits also indicate boards' failure to understand how to improve performance and craft coherent performance improvement strategies (National Health Board & Southern District Health Board, 2011). The boards may also lack the skills needed to manage DHB finances. Only under political duress and after the creation of new central agencies from 2009 have boards begun to focus on quality improvement and organisational processes, including clinical governance. This suggests that many boards have lacked the ability to think laterally about how to improve local services, including the exploration of international trends and experiences that may be adapted for local implementation. When a higher priority is given to representation than to developing an integrated health care system around national goals and benchmarks it may come at the cost of achieving objectives related to the quality and integration of health care.

Should New Zealand retain elected health boards?

A central tenet of any democratic society or arrangement is that the views of the public and local communities should be incorporated into decision-making processes. Revisiting a question raised in Chapter One, some of the reasons for involving the broader public include: (1) perceived informational advantages, since managers and health professionals lack information and make decisions behind closed doors without representation (Florin and Dixon, 2004); (2) diverse community preferences need a mechanism for representation to decide on funding levels or the location of different services (Ham and Robert, 2003); (3) it improves public accountability (Fudge et al., 2008) and greater accountability may improve health outcomes through higher quality care; and (4) greater public 'ownership' or acceptance of policies and strategic directions.

There are varying degrees to which the public might participate in the activities of an entity such as a health board, as noted in Chapter One. Public involvement and control over governing boards has diminished over the years and the boards' perceived relevance has declined. The present DHBs permit only limited scope for public involvement: their primary accountability under legislation is to central government. The DHBs are far from the ideal and they offer only 'tokenistic' public participation (Arnstein, 1969).[2] Moreover, the New Zealand model allows for the government to claim victory for local success stories while deflecting responsibility for failures or controversial decisions to the local level. These issues raise the question of whether the elected board model should be retained. If so, how might it be improved; if not, what might replace it?

First, there should be greater political scrutiny and societal debate about the merits and shortcomings of the representative model and its alternatives (which we hope will be encouraged by this book). The public should be given the opportunity to review the model, perhaps in a referendum, but people would also need more information than they have now to evaluate the boards. Discussions could be informed by empirical research on whether goals are actually being met and whether the current elected DHBs make better decisions than they would if they were appointed;

---

2. We acknowledge that using Arnstein's 'ladder of participation' as a tool for measuring DHBs as facilitators of public participation is problematic as sometimes they are vehicles for top-down government control and at others for local action to reshape central government plans. However, the ladder remains a useful concept for guiding assessments of participation, including for DHBs; DHBs were intended to be vehicles for public involvement in health care planning and decision making.

whether they represent diverse community preferences; and whether elected boards' health services are higher in quality. To ensure boards fulfil their functions and have the capacity for leadership, board members should have a comprehensive knowledge of health care. Where there are gaps, we need to think about the training that would improve the boards' capacity. An elected board masquerading as corporate-style governance may be controlled mainly by staff, which means boards will not direct and provide adequate oversight. In this situation, the full-time staff or chief executive drives the activities and thinking of the board.

If the model is to be retained, there are options for improvement, depending on the focus of health policy and the stated aims for boards. A realist position suggests that the elected members currently provide limited accountability and benefits to the general public, but the public may want some democratic control. One of our family members challenged us during the writing of this book: without an elected board, who would fight for someone who has been poorly treated? However, that role is more powerful when elections are *competitive*. To increase the competitiveness of elections New Zealand could reduce the number of elected members. Two or three elected members out of the present eleven could provide a sharper focus for candidates through increasing competition for votes and seats on boards. Voters would have fewer members to elect, which would make it easier to identify them as representatives. Coupled with this change would be clarification of elected and appointed board member roles. The specific role of elected members could be to facilitate public opinion being consulted and heard. The focus for appointed members could be on planning, operating, and improving the health services in the region and nationally. Clearly delineated roles and responsibilities under a legislative framework could also reduce disagreements between the elected and appointed members.

The idea of reducing the number of elected members is based on a realist view of the board system and requires moving away from more sentimental notions of geography and locality. A related question is whether national decisions, such as how much funding is allocated to health, are more important than local decisions about services. Traditionally, the model of elected boards was organised around hospitals in communities and disaggregated geographic areas, but our survey shows these were sometimes more historical accident than design. New Zealand does have some unique geographic features and a dispersed population, but this must be balanced against the fact that a small country has neither the financial resources of a larger population, nor the geographic size, to justify duplication of effort. History suggests that parochialism tends to be the default, if we are left to our own devices, but it might make us all worse off.

A second reason for reconsidering geography is that New Zealanders are more homogeneous in terms of their views about health services than most people realise: geography is not destiny in New Zealand; in comparing any two regions we would find (on average) that individuals' values are more similar compared to people in the same country elsewhere in the world. For example, a random selection of residents from Utah and California would show stark differences in opinions on subsidised health care for the poor, or support for making health insurance mandatory. Surveys suggest that most New Zealanders, no matter where they live, support having a public health system that is accessible and that provides quality care.

The issue of geography speaks to the question of the scale of representation. The number of boards could be reduced through mergers; for example, in the Auckland and Wellington areas and elsewhere. The right number is likely to be somewhere between the four regional health authorities of the 1990s and the twenty boards of the present. Contiguous DHBs could be encouraged (with incentives from central government) to form alliances, creating larger areas and economies of scale.[3] A larger scale may also allow greater focus on the kinds of skills necessary to provide oversight of the health care system. At present DHB members receive only limited training, yet they are expected to govern large, complex organisations. They are responsible for the expenditure of almost one in five taxpayer dollars spent by the government on public services. Board members need comprehensive training in all aspects of health care delivery and governance, comparable to that which many professional company directors seeking accreditation receive. As studies show, hospitals with boards trained in quality improvement provide higher quality health care (Jha and Epstein, 2010); DHBs should receive routine and ongoing training and their performance on various quality indicators should be monitored.

---

3. As noted in Chapter Eight, the post-2008 period has seen an emphasis on regional alliances between DHBs with the New Zealand Public Health and Disability Amendment Act 2010 mandating this. Of course, a potential disadvantage of regionalisation and fewer DHBs is a reduction in local capacity to drive change. Other changes outlined in Chapter Eight, such as creation of the Health Quality and Safety Commission, should offset this with their focus on stimulating local innovations designed to improve services and patient safety.

What are the alternatives to the existing DHB model? The period of appointed boards in New Zealand's health system through the 1990s created a legacy of distaste for that model. Given two stark options (democracy or markets), the public is bound to choose democracy. Appointed boards became associated with threats to the 'public' health service that has been symbolic of the equal and caring society that New Zealanders traditionally aspire to. But the boards appointed in the 1990s were created under a very different policy framework and set of assumptions. As argued in Chapter Two, the macro policy framework in every country sets the parameters for these larger issues, such as the role of public and private finance in a system. It all depends on how the principles are defined nationally; appointed boards can work effectively when carefully constructed and provided with reasonable goals, with many local and international examples to learn from.

In a country of New Zealand's size, having adequate representation at the national level may be more important, whether through national elections or through citizen appointees to national boards. Many appointed boards provide public and specialised clinical input that impacts on the national policy framework. Health sector examples include the National Health Committee, which has had clinical, research and community leaders since the 1990s, the National Health Board, the IT Health Board and the Health Quality and Safety Commission. With the exception of the National Health Committee, from 2009 these boards were largely comprised of health professionals with backgrounds in leadership. They follow a model of clinical governance based on management–clinician partnerships and cooperation between health professionals whose aim is to improve the health system.

At the national level, the Pharmaceutical Management Agency of New Zealand (known as Pharmac, which makes purchasing decisions related to pharmaceuticals) is another model. Pharmac's main board consults with a consumer board in order to gauge public opinion. The consumer board members are appointed from the community. Usually, members have many years of community service in different roles, and a good understanding of Pharmac's function as national drug buyer. The National Institute for Health and Clinical Excellence (NICE) in Britain uses a similar approach.

Albert O. Hirschman argues that markets tend to be governed by consumers who can exit, whereas voice is usually needed to make changes in politics and the public sector (Hirschman, 1970). While there is considerable wisdom in his theory, governance contains a mix of these qualities. A high quality accessible public health service requires that we see the world as more nuanced. We need both aspects: voice, so that individuals have some representation, and mechanisms providing for leadership that aims for the highest level of service responsiveness to its consumers.

References

CHAPTER ONE. Democratic governance and health: an introduction

1926. Defended by Minister: Board System a Well-tried Institution. *Evening Post*, 4 May, 8.

ARNOLD, R.D. 1990. *The Logic of Congressional Action*. New Haven, Yale University Press.

ARNSTEIN, S. 1969. A Ladder of Participation. Journal of the American Institute of Planners, 216–223.

ASHWIN, S.B. 1956. Financial Problems of Local Government. In: POLASCHEK, R.J. (ed.) Local Government in New Zealand. Wellington, New Zealand Institute of Public Administration.

BLOOMFIELD, G.T. 1984. New Zealand: A Handbook of Historical Statistics. Boston, GK Hall and Co.

BOHMER, R. 2010a. Leadership with a Small 'l'. BMJ, 340.

BOHMER, R.M.J. 2010b. Fixing Health Care on the Front Lines. *Harvard Business Review*, 88, 62–69.

BRISTOL ROYAL INFIRMARY INQUIRY 2001. *Learning from Bristol: The Report of the Public Inquiry into Children's Heart Surgery at the Bristol Royal Infirmary 1984–1995*. London, Stationary Office.

BRUNTON, W. 1983. Hostages to History. *New Zealand Health Review*, 3.

BUSH, G. 1992. Local Government: Politics and Pragmatism. *In:* GOLD, H. (ed.) *New Zealand Politics in Perspective (Third Edition)*. Auckland, Longman Paul.

CARTWRIGHT, S. 1988. *The Report of the Cervical Cancer Inquiry*. Auckland, Government Printing Office.

CONDLIFFE, J.B. 1959. *The Welfare State in New Zealand*. London, Ruskin House, George Allen and Unwin, Ltd.

CRAWFORD, M. J., RUTTER, D., MANLEY, C., WEAVER, T., BHUI, K., FULOP,

N. & TYRER, P. 2002. Systematic Review of Involving Patients in the Planning and Development of Health Care. *British Medical Journal*, 325, 1263–1267.

DAVIS, P., LAY-YEE, R., BRIANT, R., ALI, W., SCOTT, A. & SCHUG, S. 2002. Adverse Events in New Zealand Public Hospitals 1: Occurrence and Impact. *New Zealand Medical Journal*, 115 1167.

DEPARTMENT OF HEALTH 1961–1988. Hospital Statistics.

DEPARTMENT OF HEALTH 1973. Memo to Caucus Committees on Health on constitutional issues regarding hospital boards and regional Health Authorities, 12 December. *Restructuring the Health Service – Caucus Committee*. Wellington, National Archives. ABQU W4415 341-6 50261.

DEPARTMENT OF HEALTH 1975. *A Health Service for New Zealand*, Wellington, Government Printer.

DEPARTMENT OF HEALTH 2000. *An Organisation with a Memory. Report of an expert group on learning from adverse events in the NHS*. London, Department of Health.

FLORIN, D. & DIXON, J. 2004. Public Involvement in Health Care. *British Medical Journal*, 328, 159–161.

FUDGE, N., WOLFE, C.D.A. & MCKEVITT, C. 2008. Assessing the Promise of User Involvement in Health Service Development: Ethnographic Study. *British Medical Journal*, 336, 313–317.

GAULD, R. 2000. Big Bang and the Policy Prescription: Health Care Meets the Market in New Zealand. *Journal of Health Politics, Policy and Law*, 25, 815–844.

GAULD, R. 2001. *Revolving Doors: New Zealand's Health Reforms*, Wellington, Institute of Policy Studies and Health Services Research Centre.

GAULD, R. 2009. *The New Health Policy*. Maidenhead, Open University Press.

GAULD, R. 2010. Are Elected Health Boards an Effective Mechanism for Public Participation in Health Service Governance? *Health Expectations*, 13, 369–378.

GOOLD, M. & CAMPBELL, A. 1987. *Strategies and Styles: The Role of the Centre in Managing Diversified Corporations*. Cambridge, Basil Blackwell.

HAM, C. & ROBERT, G. (eds.) 2003. *Reasonable Rationing: International Experience of Priority Setting in Health Care*. Buckingham, Open University Press.

HEGGIE, E.G. 1969. Organizing for Health. *In:* LATIMER, R.J. (ed.) *Health Administration in New Zealand*. Wellington: New Zealand Institute of Public Administration.

HOGG, C.N. 2007. Patient and Public Involvement: What Next for the NHS? *Health Expectations: An International Journal of Public Participation in Health Care and Health Policy*, 10, 129–38.

IMMERGUT, E.M. 1992. *Health Politics: Interests and Institutions in Western Europe*. Cambridge, Cambridge University Press.

INSTITUTE OF MEDICINE 2000. *To Err is Human: Building a Safer Health System*. Washington, D.C., National Academy Press.

IRVINE, D. 1999. The Performance of Doctors: The New Professionalism. *The Lancet*, 353, 1174–1177.

IRVINE, D. 2005. GMC and the Future of Revalidation: Patients, Professionalism, and Revalidation. *British Medical Journal*, 330, 1265–1268.

KLEIN, R. 1996. 'Self-inventing Institutions: Institutional Design and the U.K. Welfare State'. *In:* GOODIN, R.E. (ed.) *The Theory of Institutional Design.* New York, Cambridge University Press.

LANE, J.E. 1995. *The Public Sector: Concepts, Models and Approaches.* London, Sage.

LAUGESEN, M. 2005. Why Some Market Reforms Lack Legitimacy in Health Care. *Journal of Health Politics, Policy and Law,* 30, 1065–100.

LEAPE, L., LAWTHERS, A.G., BRENNAN, T.A. & JOHNSON, W.G. 1993. Preventing Medical Injury. *Quality Review Bulletin,* 19, 144–149.

LEWIS, G.H., VAITHIANATHAN, R., HOCKEY, P.M., HIRST, G. & BAGIAN, J.P. 2011. Counterheroism, Common Knowledge, and Ergonomics: Concepts from Aviation that could Improve Patient Safety. *Milbank Quarterly,* 89, 4–38.

LINDBLOM, C. 1959. The Science of Muddling Through. *Public Administration Review,* 19, 79–88.

LITVA, A., CANVIN, K., SHEPHERD, M., JACOBY, A. & GABBAY, M. 2009. Lay Perceptions of the Desired Role and Type of User Involvement in Clinical Governance. *Health Expectations,* 12, 81–91.

LITVA, A., COAST, J., DONOVAN, J., EYLES, J., SHEPHERD, M., TACCHI, J., ABELSON, J. & MORGAN, K. 2002. 'The Public is Too Subjective': Public Involvement at Different Levels of Health-Care Decision Making. *Social Science & Medicine,* 54, 1825–1837.

LOCAL GOVERNMENT ASSOCIATION HEALTH COMMISSION 2008. *Who's Accountable for Health? LGA Health Commission Final Report,* London, Local Government Association.

MARTIN, J. 1991. Devolution and Decentralisation. *In:* BOSTON, J., JOHN MARTIN, JUNE PALLOT, PAT WALSH (ed.) *Reshaping the State: New Zealand's Bureaucratic Revolution.* Auckland, Oxford University Press.

MULGAN, R.G. 1984. *Democracy and Power in New Zealand: A Study of New Zealand Politics.* Auckland, Oxford University Press.

MULLEY, A.G. 2009. Inconvenient truths about supplier induced demand and unwarranted variation in medical practice. *BMJ,* 339, b4073.

NATIONAL ARCHIVES Restructuring the Health Service – Special Committee on Health Services – Organisation and Administration.

OECD 2009. *Health at a Glance 2009.* Paris, Organisation for Economic Cooperation and Development.

PERROW, C. 1986. *Complex Organizations: A Critical Essay.* New York, Random House.

PIERSON, P. 1994. *Dismantling the Welfare State?* New York, Cambridge University Press.

PIERSON, P. 2002. Increasing Returns, Path Dependence, and the Study of Politics. *American Political Science Review,* 94, 251–267.

QUALITY IMPROVEMENT COMMITTEE 2009. *Sentinel and Serious Events in New Zealand Hospitals 2007–2008.* Wellington, The Quality Improvement Committee.

RHODES, R.A.W. 1997. *Understanding Governance: Policy Networks, Governance, Reflexivity and Accountability.* Buckingham, Open University Press.

SCALLY, G. & DONALDSON, L. 1998. Clinical Governance and the Drive for Quality Improvement in the New NHS in England. *British Medical Journal*, 317, 61–65.

SHIPMAN INQUIRY 2004. *Fifth Report – Safeguarding Patients: Lessons from the Past – Proposals for the Future.* London, The Shipman Inquiry.

SMITH, P. C., MOSSIALOS, E., PAPANICOLAS, I. & LEATHERMAN, S. (eds.) 2009. *Performance Measurement for Health System Improvement: Experiences, Challenges and Prospects.* Cambridge, Cambridge University Press.

STATISTICS NEW ZEALAND 1951. New Zealand Yearbook 1950–1951. Wellington.

THOMAS, E.J., STUDDERT, D.M., BURSTIN, H.R., ORAV, E.J., ZEENA, T., WILLIAMS, E.J., HOWARD, K.M., WEILER, P.C. & BRENNAN, T.A. 2000. Incidence and Types of Adverse Events and Negligent Care in Utah and Colorado. *Medical Care*, 38, 247–249.

THORLBY, R., LEWIS, R. & DIXON, J. 2008. *Should Primary Care Trusts Be Made More Accountable Locally?* London, King's Fund.

VINCENT, C., NEALE, G. & WOLOSHYNOWYCH, M. 2001. Adverse Events in British Hospitals: Preliminary Retrospective Record Review. *British Medical Bulletin*, 322, 517–519.

WAIT, S. & NOLTE, E. 2006. Public Involvement in Policies in Health: Exploring their Conceptual Basis. *Health Economics, Policy, and Law*, 1, 149–162.

WENNBERG, J. E. 2002. Unwarranted variations in healthcare delivery: implications for academic medical centres. *BMJ*, 325, 961–4.

WILSFORD, D. 1994. Path Dependency, or Why History Makes it Difficult but Not Impossible to Reform Health Systems in a Big Way. *Journal of Public Policy*, 14, 251–283.

WILSON, R.M., RUNCIMAN, W.B., GIBBERD, R.W., HARRISON, B.T., NEWBY, B.T. & HAMILTON, J.D. 1995. The Quality in Australian Health Care Study. *Medical Journal of Australia*, 163, 458–471.

CHAPTER TWO. Cross-national models of health system governance

ASHFORD, D.E. 1986. *The Emergence of the Welfare States.* Oxford & New York, Blackwell.

AUSTRALIAN GOVERNMENT 2010. *A National Health and Hospitals Network for Australia's Future: Delivering the Reforms.* Canberra, Commonwealth of Australia.

AUSTRALIAN GOVERNMENT 2011. *Improving Primary Health Care for All Australians.* Canberra, Commonwealth of Australia.

BATTISTELLA, R.M. & CHESTER, T.E. 1973. Reorganization of the National Health Service: Background and Issues in England's Quest for a Comprehensive-Integrated Planning and Delivery System. *The Milbank Memorial Fund Quarterly. Health and Society*, 489–530.

BLANK, R.H. & BURAU, V. 2010. *Comparative Health Policy (Third Edition).* Houndmills, Palgrave Macmillan.

BOYCHUK, T. 1999. *The Making and Meaning of Hospital Policy in the United States and Canada.* Ann Arbor, University of Michigan Press.

BRIDGMAN, R.F. & ROEMER, M.I. 1973. *Hospital Legislation and Hospital Systems.* Geneva, World Health Organization.

CALLTORP, J. 1999. Priority Setting in Health Policy in Sweden and a Comparison with Norway. *Health Policy,* 50, 1–22.

CHAUDRY, B., WANG, J., WU, S., MAGLIONE, M., MOJICA, W., ROTH, E., MORTON, S. & SHEKELLE, P. 2006. Systematic Review: Impact of Health Information Technology on Quality, Efficiency, and Costs of Medical Care. *Annals of Internal Medicine,* 144, 742–752.

GAULD, R. 2004. One Step Forward, One Step Back? Restructuring, Evolving Policy and Information Technology and Management in the New Zealand Health Sector. *Government Information Quarterly,* 21, 125–142.

GAULD, R. (ed.) 2005. *Comparative Health Policy in the Asia-Pacific.* Maidenhead: Open University Press.

GAULD, R. 2010. Are Elected Health Boards an Effective Mechanism for Public Participation in Health Service Governance? *Health Expectations,* 13, 369–378.

GRAY, G. 1991. *Federalism and Health Policy: The Development of Health Systems in Canada and Australia.* Toronto, University of Toronto Press.

HEALY, J,. & MCKEE M. 2002. The Role and Functions of Hospitals. *In:* MCKEE, M. & HEALY, J. (eds.) Hospitals in a Changing Europe. Buckingham, Open University Press.

HJORTSBERG, C. & GHATNEKAR, O. 2001. *Sweden: Health Care Systems in Transition.* Copenhagen: European Observatory on Health Care Systems.

HOGG, C.N.L. 2007. Patient and Public Involvement: What Next for the NHS? *Health Expectations,* 10, 129–138.

KLARMAN, H.E. 1976. National Policies and Local Planning for Health Services. *The Milbank Memorial Fund Quarterly. Health and Society,* 54, 1–28.

LANCRY, P.J. & SANDIER, S. 1999. Rationing Health Care in France. *Health Policy,* 50, 23–38.

LEWIS, S. J., KOURI, D., ESTABROOKS, C., DICKINSON, H., DUTCHAK, J., WILLIAMS, I., MUSTARD, C. & HURLEY, J. 2001. Devolution to Democratic Health Authorities in Sashtchewan: An Interim Report. *Canadian Medical Association Journal,* 164, 343–347.

LOCAL GOVERNMENT ASSOCIATION HEALTH COMMISSION 2008. *Who's Accountable for Health? LGA Health Commission Final Report.* London, Local Government Association.

LOMAS, J., WOODS, J. & VEENSTRA, G. 1997a. Devolving Authority for Health Care in Canada's Provinces: 1. An Introduction to the Issues. *Canadian Medical Association Journal,* 156, 371–377.

LOMAS, J., WOODS, J. & VEENSTRA, G. 1997b. Devolving Authority for Health Care in Canada's Provinces: 4. Emerging Issues and Prospects. *Canadian Medical Association Journal,* 156, 817–823.

MARMOR, T., FREEMAN, R. & OKMA, K. (eds.) 2009. *Comparative Studies and the Politics of Modern Medical Care.* New Haven, Yale University Press.

MCKEE, M. & HEALY, J. 2002. *Hospitals in a Changing Europe*. Buckingham, Open University Press.

OECD 2009. *OECD Health Data*. Paris, Organisation for Economic Cooperation and Development.

OECD 2010. *Health Systems Institutional Characteristics: A Survey of 29 OECD Countries*. Paris, Organisation for Economic Cooperation and Development.

OKMA, K. (ed.) 2010. *Six Countries, Six Reform Models: The Healthcare Reform Experience of Israel, the Netherlands, New Zealand, Singapore, Switzerland and Taiwan*. Singapore, World Scientific Publishers.

PEARSON, D.A. 1976. The Concept of Regionalized Personal Health Services in the United States 1920–1955. In: SAWARD, E.W. (ed.) *The Regionalization of Personal Health Services*. Published for the Milbank Memorial Fund by Prodist.

PEARSON, D.A. & ABERNETHY, D.S. 1980. A Qualitative Assessment of Previous Efforts to Contain Hospital Costs. *Journal of Health Politics, Policy and Law,* 5, 120–141.

ROEMER, M.I. 1976. *Health Care Systems in World Perspective*. Ann Arbor, Health Administration Press.

ROLAND, M. & ROSEN, R. 2011. English NHS Embarks on Controversial and Risky Market-style Reforms in Health Care. *New England Journal of Medicine,* 364, 360–366.

RUBEL, E.J. 1976. Implementing the National Health Planning and Resources Development Act of 1974. *Public Health Reports,* 91, 3.

RUGGIE, M. 1996. *Realignments in the Welfare State: Health Policy in the United States, Britain, and Canada*. New York, Columbia University Press.

SALTMAN, R.B., BANKAUSKAITE, V. & VRANGBAEK, K. (eds.) 2007. *Decentralization in Health Care: Strategies and Outcomes*. Maidenhead, Open University Press.

SAX, S. 1984. *A Strife of Interests: Politics and Policies in Australian Health Services*. Sydney, Allen & Unwin.

SCOTTISH GOVERNMENT 2009. Elected Health Boards Get Go-Ahead. Press release 12 March. Edinburgh, The Scottish Government.

SMITH, D.B. 2005. The Politics of Racial Disparities: Desegregating the Hospitals in Jackson, Mississippi. *Milbank Quarterly,* 83, 247–269.

THE ECONOMIST 2011. Who are the world's biggest employers? *The Economist,* 12 September.

TUOHY, C.J. 1999. *Accidental Logics: The Dynamics of Change in the Health Care Arena in the United States, Britain, and Canada*. New York, Oxford University Press.

WEBSTER, C. 1998. *The NHS: A Political History*. Oxford, Oxford University Press.

CHAPTER THREE. The creation of universal health care 1925 to 1960

1924. For All Classes. *Evening Post,* 5 December.

1925. Payment for Hospital Doctors. *NZ Truth,* June, 5.

1926a. Defended by Minister: Board System a Well-tried Institution. *Evening Post,* 4 May, 8.

1926b. General Hospitals. *Evening Post*, 26 August, 15.

1928. Hospital System: Dominion Survey. *Evening Post*, 30 March.

1932a. *Evening Post*. 9 June, 12.

1932b. Day in Parliament. *Evening Post*. 23 November, 6.

1932c. Diverse Views: Dr. Begg's Scheme, Hospital Board System. *Evening Post*, 10 June, 12.

1932d. Hospital Reform. *Evening Post*, 29 January, 8.

1932e. Hospital Reform: Economies Urged. *Evening Post*, 28 January, 12.

1932f. The Hospitals. *Evening Post*, 23 November, 7.

1932g. The Hospitals. *Evening Post*, 18 November, 11.

1932h. The Hospitals: Amending Bill Protracted Debate. *Evening Post*, 30 November, 9.

1932i. House of Representatives. *Evening Post*, 17 November, 12.

1932j. National Economies. *Ellesmere Guardian*, 4 October, 7.

1933. No Hasty Action Amalgamation Scheme: Hospital Districts. *Evening Post*, 24 March, 9.

1936. The Hospitals. *Evening Post*, 14 October.

ALEXANDER TURNBULL LIBRARY 1952a. Memo from John Cairney, Director General of Health to John Marshall. MS Papers 1403 Folder 23:2, Sir John Marshall Collection.

ALEXANDER TURNBULL LIBRARY 1952b. Memo to the Minister of Health from CA Taylor for the Director General. Sir John Marshall Collection, MS Papers 1403 Folder 23:2.

ALEXANDER TURNBULL LIBRARY n.d. Unsigned paper on the Reorganisation of the Hospital System. Sir John Marshall Collection, MS Papers 1403 Folder 23:2.

BLOOMFIELD, G.T. 1984. *New Zealand, A Handbook of Historical Statistics*, Boston, MA, G.K. Hall.

BOLITHO, D.G. 1979. *The Response of the New Zealand Medical Profession to the Introduction of Social Security*. Wellington, Victoria University of Wellington.

CHAPMAN, R.M. 1962. The General Result. *In:* CHAPMAN, R.M. (ed.) *New Zealand Politics in Action: The 1960 General Election*. London, Oxford University Press.

CHAPMAN, R.M. 1991. From Labour to National. *In:* OLIVER, W.H., RICE, G. & WILLIAMS, B.R. (eds.) *The Oxford History of New Zealand (Second Edition)*. Auckland, Oxford University Press.

CONSULTATIVE COMMITTEE ON HOSPITAL REFORM 1953. *Report of the Consultative Committee on Hospital Reform*, Wellington.

DEPARTMENT OF HEALTH 1969. *A Review of Hospital & Related Services in New Zealand*. Wellington, Department of Health.

DEPARTMENT OF HEALTH 1975. *A Health Service for New Zealand*. Wellington, Government Printer.

DOW, D. A. 1995. *Safeguarding the Public Health: A History of the New Zealand Department of Health*. Wellington, Victoria University Press.

FRASER, G. 1984. An Examination of Factors in the Development of New

Zealand's Health System. *In:* WILKES, C. & SHIRLEY, I. (eds.) *In the Public Interest: Health, Work and Housing in New Zealand Society.* Auckland, Benton Ross.

HANSARD 1935. Parliamentary Paper H-30: Departmental Committee on National Compulsory Superannuation and Health Insurance. Wellington, House of Representatives.

HANSON, E. 1980. *The Politics of Social Security: The 1938 Act and Some Later Developments.* Auckland, Auckland University Press.

HARRIS, P., LEVINE, S., CLARK, M., MARTIN, J. & MCLEAY, E.M. 1992. *The New Zealand Politics Source Book.* Palmerston North, Dunmore Press.

HAWKE, G.R. 1984. *The Making of New Zealand: An Economic History.* New York, Cambridge University Press.

HAY, I. 1989. *The Caring Commodity: The Provision of Health Care in New Zealand.* Auckland, Oxford University Press.

HEGGIE, E.G. 1969. Organizing for Health. *In:* LATIMER, R.J. (ed.) *Health Administration in New Zealand.* Wellington, New Zealand Institute of Public Administration.

HON. GEORGE F. GAIR 1980. *The Equitable Distribution of Finance to Hospital Boards: A Report to the Minister of Health.* Wellington, Advisory Committee on Hospital Board Funding.

IMMERGUT, E.M. 1992. *Health Politics: Interests and Institutions in Western Europe.* Cambridge, Cambridge University Press.

INTERNATIONAL LABOUR OFFICE 1936. Record of Proceedings Geneva: League of Nations.

LOVELL-SMITH, J.B. 1966. *The New Zealand Doctor and the Welfare State.* Auckland, Blackwood & Janet Paul.

MARSHALL, J. 1983. *Memoirs: Volume One, 1912 to 1960.* Auckland, Collins.

MILNE, R.S. 1966. *Political Parties in New Zealand.* Oxford, Clarendon Press.

NATIONAL ARCHIVES 1921–1941. Report by the Executive of the Hospital Boards' Association of New Zealand. ADBZ 1 1320 11290.

NATIONAL ARCHIVES 1936. Report: Nash Papers. Folio 11111.

NATIONAL ARCHIVES 1936–1937. Social Security National Health Insurance Investigation Replies to Questionnaire. AAFB 1 1378 13989.

NATIONAL ARCHIVES 1937a. Evidence tendered by the B.M.A. to the NHIIC. Nash Papers 1007 0002.

NATIONAL ARCHIVES 1937b. Notes of Conference Held Between Members of the British Medical Association and the Hon. W. Nash and Hon. P. Fraser. Nash Papers 1007 0041-54.

NATIONAL ARCHIVES 1938a. Ancient Order of Foresters to Minister of Finance. Nash Papers 1013 0228.

NATIONAL ARCHIVES 1938b. New Zealand Counties Association Memorandum on Social Security. Nash Papers Folio 1017 0237.

NATIONAL ARCHIVES 1938c. New Zealand Farmers' Union Statement made by the Dominion President, Mr. W.W. Mulholland to the Select Committee on National Health and Superannuation 1017 0255.

NATIONAL ARCHIVES 1950a. Social Security – Newspaper Cuttings: 1950–1971, *The Dominion*. ABQU H 206-5 40792.

NATIONAL ARCHIVES 1950b. Social Security – Newspaper Cuttings: 1950–1971, *The New Zealand Observer*. ABQU 206-5 40792.

NATIONAL ARCHIVES 1950c. Social Security – Newspaper Cuttings: 1950–1971, *Southern Cross*. ABQU 206-5 40792.

NATIONAL ARCHIVES 1950d. Social Security – Newspaper Cuttings: 1950–1971, *The Standard*. ABQU 206-5 40792.

NATIONAL ARCHIVES 1953a. Clutha Branch of Federated Farmers letter. AAFB 197-4 26037.

NATIONAL ARCHIVES 1953b. Consultative Committee on Hospital Reform Submissions – Wellington Submissions, Department of Health, Fourth Statement. ABQU W4415 608.

NATIONAL ARCHIVES 1953c. Consultative Committee on Hospital Reform Submissions – Wellington Submissions, Department of Health, Sixth Statement. ABQU W4415 608.

NATIONAL ARCHIVES 1953d. Consultative Committee on Hospital Reform Submissions – Wellington Submissions, Stratford Hospital Board Submission. ABQU W4415 608.

NATIONAL ARCHIVES 1953e. Consultative Committee on Hospital Reform Submissions – Wellington Submissions, Submissions from the New Zealand Registered Nurses' Association, Private Hospitals Association, and the British Medical Association. ABQU W4415 608.

NATIONAL ARCHIVES 1953f. Consultative Committee on Hospital Reform Submissions – Wellington Submissions. Submission from Wellington Hospital Board, Submission from the Hawera Hospital Board, Submission from the Dannevirke Hospital Board. ABQU W4415.

NATIONAL ARCHIVES 1953g. Consultative Committee on Hospital Reform Submissions, Dunedin Sitting: Various Submissions. ABQU W4415 608.

NATIONAL ARCHIVES 1953h. Consultative Committee on Hospital Reform Submissions, Submission from Thames Hospital Board, Auckland Submissions. ABQU W4415 609.

NATIONAL ARCHIVES 1953i. Letter from Secretary of Balclutha Businessman's Association. AAFB H1 54/197/4 26037.

NATIONAL ARCHIVES 1953j. Social Security – Newspaper Cuttings: 1950–1971, Taranaki Daily News. ABQU 206-5 40792.

NATIONAL ARCHIVES n.d. Report: Nash Papers: 1022. Folio 00004.

NEW ZEALAND HOUSE OF REPRESENTATIVES 1975. *A Health Service for New Zealand: Presented to the House of Representatives*. Wellington, Government Printer.

NEW ZEALAND MEDICAL ASSOCIATION n.d. Jamieson Papers Collection.

NORTH, D.C. 1981. *Structure and Change in Economic History*. New York, Norton.

OLIVER, W.H. 1977. The Origins and Growth of the Welfare State. *In:* TRLIN, A. D. (ed.) *Social Welfare and New Zealand Society*. Wellington, Methuen Publications.

STATISTICS NEW ZEALAND 1958. *New Zealand Yearbook 1958–1959.* Wellington, Government Printer.

STATISTICS NEW ZEALAND 1968. *New Zealand Yearbook 1968–1969,* Wellington, Government Printer.

WIGGLESWORTH, S. 1954. *The Depression and the Election of 1935.* Masters thesis, Victoria University of Wellington.

CHAPTER FOUR. Rational planning meets democratic forces

BASSETT, M. 1976. *The Third Labour Government: A Personal History.* Palmerston North, Dunmore Press.

BROOKES, R.H. The New Proposals. *In:* COOPER, M.H. & SHANNON, P.T. (eds.) A New Health Service for New Zealand, 11–13 November 1977, Department of University Extension, University of Otago.

BRUNTON, W. 1983. Hostages to History. *New Zealand Health Review,* 3.

CONEY, S. 1993. Health Organisations. *In:* ELSE, A. (ed.) *Women Together: A History of Women's Organisations in New Zealand.* Wellington: Historical Branch, Department of Internal Affairs and Daphne Brasell Press.

DEPARTMENT OF HEALTH 1969. *A Review of Hospital & Related Services in New Zealand.* Wellington, Department of Health.

DEPARTMENT OF HEALTH 1975. *A Health Service for New Zealand.* Wellington, Government Printer.

DEPARTMENT OF HEALTH 1982. Health Services Reorganisation: A Discussion Document.

DEPARTMENT OF HEALTH: DIVISION OF HOSPITALS 1967–1984. Hospital Statistics of New Zealand, Hospital Management Data. *In:* NATIONAL HEALTH STATISTICS CENTRE: DEPT. OF HEALTH (ed.) various ed.

DIXON, C.W. 1969. Regional Medical Planning in New Zealand. *New Zealand Medical Journal,* 69, 371–4.

EAGLES, J. & JAMES, C. 1973. *The Making of a New Zealand Prime Minister.* Wellington, Cheshire Press.

FREIDSON, E. 1970. *Professional Dominance: The Social Structure of Medical Care.* New York, Aldine.

HANSARD 1973. *New Zealand Parliamentary Debates.* Wellington, House of Representatives.

HANSARD 1977. *New Zealand Parliamentary Debates.* Wellington, House of Representatives.

HARRIS, P., LEVINE, S.I., CLARK, M., MCLEAY, E.M. & MARTIN, J.E. 1992. *The New Zealand Politics Source Book.* Palmerston North, Dunmore Press.

HON. GEORGE F. GAIR 1980. *The Equitable Distribution of Finance to Hospital Boards: A Report to the Minister of Health.* Wellington Advisory Committee on Hospital Board Funding.

JACK, P.A. & ROBB, J.H. 1977. Social Welfare Policies: Development and Patterns since 1945. *In:* TRLIN, A.D. (ed.) *Social Welfare and New Zealand Society.* Wellington, Methuen Publications.

KINGDON, J.W. 1995. *Agendas, Alternatives and Public Policies.* New York, Harper Collins.

KIRK, N.E. 1975. The Philosophy of the Labour Party. *In:* LEVINE, S. I. (ed.) *New Zealand Politics: A Reader.* Melbourne, Cheshire Publishing.

MANZ 7 April 1975. *RE: Letter to W.J. Treadwell.*

MARTIN, J. 1991. Devolution and Decentralisation. *In:* BOSTON, J., JOHN MARTIN, JUNE PALLOT, PAT WALSH (ed.) *Reshaping the State: New Zealand's Bureaucratic Revolution.* Auckland, Oxford University Press.

MARTIN, J. 1997. Interview with John Martin. Wellington.

MEDICAL ASSOCIATION OF NEW ZEALAND 1971. Number 163. *News and Views.* New Zealand.

NATIONAL ARCHIVES. ABQU W4452 53–53.

NATIONAL ARCHIVES Memo to State Services Commission from N. Callow for Permanent Head. Wellington: AAFB H W2262 53 51894.

NATIONAL ARCHIVES Various Press Clippings. Wellington: ABQU WF4415 170-2-9 50670.

NATIONAL ARCHIVES 1969a. Letter from New Zealand National Party to Minister of Health. Wellington: W4452 169-28-1.

NATIONAL ARCHIVES 1969b. Memo from E.G. Heggie to Dr. Thompson. Wellington: AAFB H 206-28.

NATIONAL ARCHIVES 1969–1970. Submission from the Department of Health to the Royal Commission on Social Security Paper I: (a) Administration of Health Services in New Zealand and (b) Legislative basis for payment of Medical Benefits. Wellington: AAFB W2676 36710 50 36710.

NATIONAL ARCHIVES 1971–1973. Hospital Boards: Commission of Inquiry into Hospital Services Secretariat and Staffing. W2262 5/51894.

NATIONAL ARCHIVES 1972a. COM 12/12 Submissions 81–123. Wellington: 12/12 COM.

NATIONAL ARCHIVES 1972b. Royal Commissions Series: COM 12/9; COM 12/8; COM 12/10 Wellington: 12/8-10 COM.

NATIONAL ARCHIVES 1973a. Hospital Boards: Commission of Inquiry into Hospital Services Secretariat and Staffing, Memo to SSC from N. Callow for Permanent Head. AAFB W2262 53-52-1.

NATIONAL ARCHIVES 1973b. Press Statement from the Minister of Health. Wellington: ABQU W4415 107-2-9 50670.

NATIONAL ARCHIVES 1973c. Restructuring the Health Service – Caucus Committee Memo to Caucus Committees on Health. Wellington: ABQU W4415 341-5 50261.

NATIONAL ARCHIVES 1973d. Submission Number HI48: Paper on Reform of Health Services Administration. Wellington: AAFB 625 W4415.

NATIONAL ARCHIVES 1973–1977. Submissions to Caucus Committee on Health: Submission Number HI48 From Dept. of Health to Caucus Committee. Wellington: ABQU 632 W4415 341/6 50261.

NATIONAL ARCHIVES 1974. Department of Health Waiting List Data quoted in COM 12/12. Wellington: COM 12/12.

NATIONAL ARCHIVES 1976a. Administration conveying information to the press series, 1976 Public Relations Policy for Health Department. W4415 52578.

NATIONAL ARCHIVES 1976b. Speech Notes: Dr. I. Shearer, M.P. The Dual System of Health Care. AAFB W4415 638/1.

NATIONAL ARCHIVES 1976c. Speech Notes: The Minister of Health to the Medical Superintendents' Association Conference. Wellington: AAFB W4415 638.

NATIONAL ARCHIVES 1976d. White Paper on Health: Proposed Activities During 1975–1976 by the Tourist and Publicity Department. ABQU 584 W4415 341-5 50262.

NATIONAL ARCHIVES 1978. Restructuring the Health Services – General Paper to Director General's Meeting Re: Health District Boundaries. ABQU 632 W4415 583 53064.

NATIONAL ARCHIVES 1979. Administration – Health Policies and Programmes. ABQU W4415 593 51109.

NATIONAL ARCHIVES 1980-1982. Restructuring the Health Service – Media Seminar. Wellington: ABQU 632 W4415 593 56579.

NATIONAL ARCHIVES 1982a. Memorandum for Cabinet from the Minister of Health. ABQU W4415 55354.

NATIONAL ARCHIVES 1982b. SACHSO – Legislative Apects: Notes for Visit of Minister of Health to SACHSO on 17/2/82. SACHSO W4452 1515 60631.

NATIONAL ARCHIVES 1982–1984. Restructuring the Health Service – SACHSO (Papers circulated to members) ABQU 632 W4452 1514 60637.

NATIONAL ARCHIVES 1983a. Memorandum for the Minister of Health from the Deputy Director General of Health Administration. ABQU W4415 341-17 55354.

NATIONAL ARCHIVES 1983b. Restructuring Health Services – Establishment of Area Health Boards. ABQU 632 W4415 594 55354.

NATIONAL ARCHIVES 1983c. SACHSO – Legislative Aspects (Press Release Draft). ABQU W4452 632 60631.

NATIONAL ARCHIVES n.d. Minister of Health T.M. McGuigan: Address to Men's Fellowship of St. Johns Church, Whangarei. Wellington: AAFB 638 W4415

NEW ZEALAND MEDICAL ASSOCIATION Files. 63-24-4.

NEW ZEALAND MEDICAL ASSOCIATION 1975a. Files. 63-24-3.

NEW ZEALAND MEDICAL ASSOCIATION 1975b. Letter from David Wills on behalf of Nurses Reform Association of New Zealand to Treadwell, W.J., 63-24-4.

NEW ZEALAND MEDICAL ASSOCIATION 1975c. Letter from the Office of the Opposition to W. Treadwell. 63-24-3.

NEW ZEALAND MEDICAL ASSOCIATION 1975d. Letter from W.J. Treadwell to Minister of Health. 63-24-4.

NEW ZEALAND MEDICAL ASSOCIATION c. 1975. Meeting Notes. Wellington, New Zealand Medical Association. 63-24-4.

NEW ZEALAND MEDICAL JOURNAL 1968a. Editorial: Medical Policy. *New Zealand Medical Journal*, 68, 33.

NEW ZEALAND MEDICAL JOURNAL 1968b. Editorial: Where Are We Going. *New Zealand Medical Journal,* 68, 545–6.

NEW ZEALAND NATIONAL PARTY 1969. *General Election Policy.* Wellington, New Zealand National Party.

OECD 1999. Health Data. Paris, Organisation for Economic Cooperation and Development.

RELMAN, A.S. 1980. The new medical-industrial complex. *New England Journal of Medicine,* 303, 963–970.

SKOCPOL, T. 1985. *Bringing the State Back In.* Cambridge, Cambridge University Press.

SOCIAL SCIENCE DATA ARCHIVES 1975. Pre-Election Survey 1975. Canberra: Social Science Data Archives, Research School of Social Sciences D0556.

TEMPLETON, I.C. & EUNSON, K. 1969. *Election '69: An Independent Survey of the New Zealand Political Scene.* Wellington, Reed.

WEST, H.G. 1981. Health Care – Present and Future. *In:* MOORE, D.J. (ed.) *The Reorganisation of the Health Services: A Tribute to Ralph Brookes.* NZ Institute of Public Administration.

CHAPTER FIVE. Inching towards marketisation, 1984 to 1990

1987a. Article. *National Business Review,* 2 October.

Eye Witness News, 1987b. Newscast. Denmark: Log TV 2.

ASHTON, T. 1992. Reform of the Health Services: Weighing Up the Costs and Benefits. *In:* BOSTON, J. & DALZIEL, P. (eds.) *The Decent Society? Essays in Response to National's Economic and Social Policies.* Auckland, Oxford University Press.

BOSTON, J. 1989. The Treasury and the Organisation of Economic Advice: Some International Comparisons. *In:* EASTON, B. (ed.) *The Making of Rogernomics.* Auckland, Auckland University Press.

BOSTON, J. 1991. The Theoretical Underpinnings of Public Sector Restructuring in New Zealand. *In:* BOSTON, J., MARTIN, J., PALLOT, J. & WALSH, P. (eds.) *Reshaping the State: New Zealand's bureaucratic revolution.* Auckland, Oxford University Press.

CLARK, L. 1987a. Douglas Losing High Ground on Health. *National Business Review,* 13 October.

CLARK, L. 1987b. No user-pays health, promises Labour. *National Business Review,* 13 August.

DAVIES, S. 1989. Health Sector Reform: The Quest for Greater Accountability. *Public Sector,* 12, 8–9.

DOUGLAS, R. 1980. *There's Got to Be a Better Way! A Practical ABC to Solving New Zealand's Major Problems.* Wellington, Fourth Estate Books.

EASTON, B. & GERRITSEN, R. 1996. Economic Reform: Parallels and Divergences. *In:* CASTLES, F. G., GERRISTEN, R. & VOWLES, J. (eds.) *The Great Experiment: Labour parties and Public Policy Transformation in Australia and New Zealand.* St. Leonards, Allen & Unwin.

ELLIS, J.W. 1998. *Voting for Markets or Marketing for Votes? The Politics of Neoliberal Economic Reform (Australia, New Zealand, Denmark).* Ph.D Dissertation, Harvard University.

EVANS, L., GRIMES, A. & WILKINSON, B. 1996. Economic Reform in New Zealand 1984–85: The Pursuit of Efficiency. *Journal of Economic Literature,* 34 1856–1902.

FRANKLIN, H. 1985. *Cul De Sac: The Question of New Zealand's Future,* Wellington, George Allen & Unwin Paperbacks/Port Nicholson Press.

GOLD, H. 1986. The Social Bases of Party Choice *In:* GOLD, H. (ed.) *New Zealand Politics in Perspective.* Auckland, Longman Paul.

GOLDFINCH, S. 2000. *Remaking New Zealand and Australian Economic Policy: Ideas, Institutions, and Policy Communities.* Washington D.C., Georgetown University Press.

JAMES, C. 1986. *The Quiet Revolution: Turbulence and Transition in Contemporary New Zealand.* Wellington, Harper Collins Publishers, Ltd.

JAMES, C. 1992. *New Territory: The Transformation of New Zealand, 1984–92.* Wellington, Bridget Williams Books.

KELSEY, J. 1996. *The New Zealand Experiment: A World Model for Structural Adjustment?* Auckland, Auckland University Press with Bridget Williams Books.

MANNION, R. 1987. Health Services Take a Cure. *Dominion Sunday Times* 6 December.

MARTIN, J. 1991. Devolution and Decentralisation. *In:* BOSTON, J., JOHN MARTIN, JUNE PALLOT, PAT WALSH (ed.) *Reshaping the State: New Zealand's Bureaucratic Revolution.* Auckland, Oxford University Press.

NAGEL, J.H. 1998. Social Choice in a Pluraltarian Democracy: The Politics of Market Liberalization in New Zealand. *British Journal of Political Science,* 28, 223–267.

NATIONAL ARCHIVES 195. Presentation by Treasury to the Board of Health Standing Committee on Allocation and Organisation. ABQU 632 W4452 403 60757.

NATIONAL ARCHIVES 1981–1986. Memo from J. Martin: Administration – Review and Development – Health Benefits, Review, Background Papers. ABQU 632 W4452 1077 61769.

NATIONAL ARCHIVES 1982–1990. Restructuring the Health Service – Restructuring of the Health Services – West Coast Administration and Personal Issues. ABQU 632 W4452 1527 71738.

NATIONAL ARCHIVES 1985a. Background Papers: *Otago Daily Times.* ABQU 632 W4452 1077 78563.

NATIONAL ARCHIVES 1985b. David Smyth talk to Health Dept Senior Personnel: 'Social Equity – A Treasury View'. ABQU 632 W4452 169-73-0-3.

NATIONAL ARCHIVES 1985c. To Minister of Health from G.C. Salmond. ABQU 632 W4452 1016 78150.

NATIONAL ARCHIVES 1985–1986. Health Benefits Review Team Report. ABQU 169-73-0-3.

NATIONAL ARCHIVES 1986a. Chairman of Board of Health Committee on

Allocation and Organisation from V.O. Sullivan, Chairman of NZ Board of Health. ABQU 632 W4452 1638 62748.

NATIONAL ARCHIVES 1986b. Memo to R. Douglas from Bassett, Health Benefits Review Background Papers. 169-73-0-3.

NATIONAL ARCHIVES 1986c. Motivations, Incentives, and Interventions in the Health Sector: Equity & Efficiency Issues, David Smyth: Treasury to the Minister of Finance. ABQU 632 W4452 1089 64416.

NATIONAL ARCHIVES 1986d. Submission Summary. ABQU W4452 632 1077 61805.

NATIONAL ARCHIVES 1987a. Address to the Hospital Boards' Association. ABQU 632 W4452 1089 64416.

NATIONAL ARCHIVES 1987b. Administration – Review and Development – Health Sector Taskforce. 632 W4452 1088 64413.

NATIONAL ARCHIVES 1987c. Administrative Review and Development of Health Benefits ABQU 632 W4452 1075 62389.

NATIONAL ARCHIVES 1987d. Briefing Notes for Ministers of Finance and Health – Meeting with consultants of the hospital and related taskforce: schedule for Thursday evening from Gordon Davies, Acting Manager Operations. ABQU 632 W4452 1090 62673.

NATIONAL ARCHIVES 1987e. Health Sector Taskforce. ABQU 632 W4452 1087 63153.

NATIONAL ARCHIVES 1987f. Health Sector Taskforce Eighth meeting of Hospital and Related Services Taskforce. ABQU 632 W4452.

NATIONAL ARCHIVES 1987g. Hospital and Related Services Taskforce. Wellington, National Archives ABQU 169-87 62745.

NATIONAL ARCHIVES 1987h. Kevin Sampson, Treasury, Comments at Workshop on Health Management. ABQU 632 W4452 1089 64416.

NATIONAL ARCHIVES 1987i. Letter to the Minister of Finance 4 February (K.B. Sampson for the Secretary to the Treasury). Wellington, National Archives ABQU W4452 632.

NATIONAL ARCHIVES 1987j. Letter to the Minister of Finance from K.B. Sampson for the Secretary to the Treasury. ABQU 632 W4452 1090 64410.

NATIONAL ARCHIVES 1987k. Memo to the Minister of Health and the Minister of Finance from the Director General of Health and the Assistant Secretary to the Treasury Health Sector Development Project; Re: Operational Approvals. WBQU 632 W4452 1090 64410.

NATIONAL ARCHIVES 1987l. Notes of a Hospital and Related Services Taskforce Meeting. ABQU 632 W44521.

NATIONAL ARCHIVES 1987m. Notes on 'Consumer' and Centrally Funded Model (70 and 71) P.J. Scott. ABQU 632 W4552 1090 64410.

NATIONAL ARCHIVES 1987n. Notes on Meeting of Hospital and Related Services Taskforce held in Auckland. ABQU 632 W4452 1087 66791.

NATIONAL ARCHIVES 1987o. Observations on Proposed Changes in the NZ Health Care System by Harold S. Luft. ABQU 632 W4452 1090 64412.

NATIONAL ARCHIVES 1987p. Points Raised at the Fifth Meeting of the Hospital and Related Services Taskforce. ABQU 632 W4452 1087 66791.

NATIONAL ARCHIVES 1987q. Points Raised at the Sixth Meeting of the Taskforce – Notes by John Scott. ABQU 632 W4452 1088 64413.

NATIONAL ARCHIVES 1987r. Points Raised at the Third Meeting of the Hospital and Related Services Taskforce. ABQU 632 W4452 1097 66791.

NATIONAL ARCHIVES 1987s. Professor A.J. Culyer, University of York on 'Reforming and Re-financing New Zealand's Health Services'. ABQU 632 W4452 62784.

NATIONAL ARCHIVES 1987t. Proposal for a Restructured Health Service. ABQU 632 W4452 1090 64412.

NATIONAL ARCHIVES 1987u. Public Hospital Services – Development of Issues, Problems, and Achievements. ABQU 632 W4452 1087 66791.

NATIONAL ARCHIVES 1987v. Roger Douglas Minister of Finance Address to the Hospital Boards' Association Biennial Conference. ABQU 632 W4452 1089 64416.

NATIONAL ARCHIVES 1987w. State Health Insurance Entitlement: Conditions and Transferability. ABQU 632 W4452 1090 64412.

NATIONAL ARCHIVES 1987x. Submission from HBA. ABQU 632 W4452 1091 64414.

NATIONAL ARCHIVES 1987y. The Supply Side Fix Draft. ABQU 632 W4452 1090 64647.

NATIONAL ARCHIVES 1987z. Telegram to Michael Bassett from Peter Cullen, Secretary, Wellington Hotel and Hospital Workers Union. ABQU 632 W4452 1090 62745.

NATIONAL ARCHIVES 1987. What do Hospitals Provide other than just care? What are Consumers' expectations? Memo to the Taskforce on Hospital and Related Services by M.E. Holman. Wellington, National Archives ABQU W4452 632 64416.

NATIONAL ARCHIVES 1987–1988a. Health Sector Taskforce. ABQU 632 W4552 1086 63540.

NATIONAL ARCHIVES 1987–1988b. Memo to Alan Gibbs, Dorothy Fraser, John Scott from Kevin Sampson. Subject Taskforce Report. ABQU 632 W4452 1090 66785.

NATIONAL ARCHIVES 1987–1988c. Royal Commission on Social Policy Briefing on Health Session on 'Choices for Health Care'. ABQU 632 W4552 1091 64414.

NATIONAL ARCHIVES 1988a. Fax to Gordon, Peter, Louise from Alan Gibbs, Re: Suggested Approach. ABQU 632 W4452 1090 64410.

NATIONAL ARCHIVES 1988b. Letter from the Wellington Hospital Board. ABQU 632 W4452 471.

NATIONAL ARCHIVES 1988c. Letter to David Lange from Alan Gibbs. ABQU 632 W4452 1090 64647.

NATIONAL ARCHIVES 1988d. Letters to consultants – Fraser, Gibbs, Scott, from Ministers of Health and Finance. ABQU 632 W4452 1090 64410.

NATIONAL ARCHIVES 1988e. Memo to Gordon Davies, from George Salmond re New Zealand Public Hospital Performance Assessment. ABQU 632 W4452 1090 64647.

NATIONAL ARCHIVES 1988f. Memo to Louise Callan from Peter Bushnell. ABQU 632 W4452 1090 64647.

NATIONAL ARCHIVES 1988g. Memo to Minister of Health from Loraine Hawkins. ABQU 632 W4452 1090 64410.

NATIONAL ARCHIVES 1988h. Minister of Finance Draft from Bevan Burgess-Exec Asst. for Minister of Finance. ABQU 632.

NATIONAL ARCHIVES 1988i. Notes of Hospital Boards' Association Meeting of Board Chairmen. ABQU 632 W4452 1090 64410.

NATIONAL ARCHIVES 1988j. Office of the Minister of Health Memorandum for Social Equity Committee. ABQU 632 W4452 1090 64647.

NATIONAL ARCHIVES 1988k. The Press: Health Sector Taskforce ABQU 632 W4452 1087 63153.

NATIONAL ARCHIVES 1988l. Response from the HBA of NZ to Unshackling the Hospitals the Report of the Hospital and Related Services Taskforce. ABQU 632 W4452 311.

NATIONAL ARCHIVES 1988m. Review of Health Benefits. Memo from Roger Douglas, Minister of Finance to the Chairman of the Cabinet Social Equity Committee. ABQU 632 W4452 1074 69863.

NATIONAL ARCHIVES 1988n. Speech from David Caygill Address to the New Zealand Medical Association Conference Gleniti Golf Club, Timaru. ABQU 632 W4452 311.

NATIONAL ARCHIVES 1988o. Working Meeting. ABQU 632 W4552 1090 64647.

NATIONAL ARCHIVES c1987. Speech from RO Douglas Minister of Finance, Address to the NZIER Members' Lunch, James Cook Hotel, Wellington. ABQU W4452 311.

NATIONAL RESEARCH BUREAU 1986. Public Perspectives of the New Zealand Health System and General Practitioners. Auckland, National Research Bureau.

NEW ZEALAND HOSPITAL & RELATED SERVICES TASKFORCE 1988. *Unshackling the Hospitals: Report*, Wellington, Government Printing Office.

NEW ZEALAND MEDICAL ASSOCIATION 1987–1988. Submission Summary to Medical Workforce Advisory Committee – NZMA, NZRMA, NZ Senior Medical Officers Association, New Zealand Association of Part-time Hospital Staff. ABQU, W4452, 632, 169-87 64412.

NEW ZEALAND MEDICAL JOURNAL. 1988. Package Poses New Questions. *New Zealand Medical Journal*, 23 November.

NEWHOUSE, J.P. 1994. Patients at Risk: Health Reform and Risk Adjustment. *Health Affairs*, 13, 132–146.

NEWHOUSE, J.P. 1996. Reimbursing Health Plans and Health Providers: Efficiency in Production Versus Selection *Journal of Economic Literature*, 34, 1236–1263.

ROBERTS, J. 1987. *Politicians, Public Servants and Public Enterprise: Restructuring the New Zealand Government Executive*. Wellington, Victoria University Press for the Institute of Policy Studies.

ROTHSCHILD, M. & STIGLITZ, J. 1976. Equilibrium in Competitive Insurance Markets: An Essay on the Economics of Imperfect Information. *Quarterly Journal of Economics*, 90, 629–649.

SCOTT, C. Health Sector Reform in New Zealand: Proceedings of Conference on Economic and Social Reform: UK–NZ Committee. 15–17 September 1989 Windsor, Victoria University.

SCOTT, C., FOUGERE, G. & MARWICK, J. 1989. *Choices for Health Care: Report of The Health Benefits Review.* Wellington, Government Printer.

CHAPTER SIX. The end of elected boards

1987. Evening Post. *Evening Post*, 26 May.

ASHTON, T. 1992. Reform of the Health Services: Weighing Up the Costs and Benefits. *In:* BOSTON, J. & DALZIEL, P. (eds.) *The Decent Society? Essays in Response to National's Economic and Social Policies.* Auckland, Oxford University Press.

ATKINSON, J. 1994. Health Reform and 'Thin' Democracy. *Political Science*, 46.

BOSTON, J., DALZIEL, P. & ST. JOHN, S. 1999. *Redesigning the Welfare State in New Zealand: Problems, Policies, Prospects.* Auckland and New York, Oxford Univerity Press.

DEPARTMENT OF PRIME MINISTER AND CABINET 1992. Report and Recommendations to the Social Services Committee on the Submissions Received on the Health and Disability Services Bill. Wellington, Deparment of Prime Minister and Cabinet.

FERGUSON, S. 1995. *The Inconvenient Realities of Health Care Reform.* Master of Arts thesis, University of Auckland.

GAULD, R. 2000. Big Bang and the Policy Prescription: Health Care Meets the Market in New Zealand. *Journal of Health Politics, Policy and Law*, 25, 815–844.

HEYLEN/TVNZ 1991. Heylen/TVNZ Poll. Wellington.

LAUGESEN, M. 2005. Why some market reforms lack legitimacy in health care. *Journal of Health Politics, Policy and Law*, 30, 1065–100.

MINISTRY OF HEALTH Health Reforms Management Group Agenda from Meeting at Vogel House. HC 28-21-0.

MINISTRY OF HEALTH Letters in response to Official Information Request. HC 28-40-0#4.

MINISTRY OF HEALTH 1990. Cabinet Strategy Committee CSC (90) M 47/7.

MINISTRY OF HEALTH 1991a. Department of Prime Minister and Cabinet to Minister of Health and Minister of Crown Health Enterprises, Re: Health Reforms Preliminary Timetable Re: announcement, Wellington.

MINISTRY OF HEALTH 1991b. Draft Amendment to CAB (90) M 45/7: Report to the Ministerial Task Force on Funding and Provision of Health Services – Draft Terms of Reference, Wellington.

MINISTRY OF HEALTH 1991c. Memorandum for Cabinet. Reform of the Funding and Provision of Health Services, 7 June. Office of the Prime Minister. Authors: Hawkins, L, Scott, C. Wellington, Ministry of Health. HC 28-28-0.

MINISTRY OF HEALTH 1991d. Memorandum for the Prime Ministerial Committee on the Reform of Social Assistance. HC 28-28-0.

MINISTRY OF HEALTH 1991e. Notes from Meeting with Minister of Health by David Smyth. HC 28-21-1.

MINISTRY OF HEALTH 1991f. Options for Social Insurance Financing of Health Annex to Memorandum for the Prime Ministerial Committee on the Reform of Social Assistance, 2. May 1991. From Rod Carr, Convenor. HC 28-28-0.

MINISTRY OF HEALTH 1991g. Scoping Paper on Core Services. HC 28 36-1.

MINISTRY OF HEALTH 1991h. Your Health and the Public Health: A Statement of Government Policy by Simon Upton. Wellington.

MINISTRY OF HEALTH 1992a. Cabinet Committee on Implementation of Social Assistance Reforms. SAR M 26/10 HC 28-14-0.

MINISTRY OF HEALTH 1992b. Draft 13: Relationship RHAs to Government. HC 28-36-2#3.

MINISTRY OF HEALTH 1992c. Fax to Patricia Danzon from Sue Begg, CS First Boston. HC 28-36-2#3.

MINISTRY OF HEALTH 1992d. Health Reforms Directorate. Wellington.

MINISTRY OF HEALTH 1992e. Health Reforms Directorate – Health Reforms – Health Care Providers Notes from meeting with Minister of Health. HC 28-21-1.

MINISTRY OF HEALTH 1992f. Memo to David Smyth, from Paul Gini on User Charges. HC 28 40-0#1.

MINISTRY OF HEALTH 1992g. Memo to User Charges Steering Committee – From Paul Gini Re: High Use Health Card Anomalies. HC 28 40-0#1.

MINISTRY OF HEALTH 1992h. Minutes of a Meeting with Birch, Upton, Luxton, Creech, WIlliamson, and O'Regan, 8 July. HC 28-14-0#2.

MINISTRY OF HEALTH 1992i. Record of Meeting of Regional Health Authority Establishment Board Chairs. HC 36-0#4.

MINISTRY OF HEALTH 1993a. Draft Work Program: HSRMU, 6 September HC 27.

MINISTRY OF HEALTH 1993b. Letter to Minister of Health, Re: Crown Health Enterprise finance from Health Sector Reform Management Unit David Newman – Chair HSRMU Advisory Committee. HC 27-00-0.

MINISTRY OF HEALTH 1993c. Meeting: Policy Guidelines Project. HC 27-00-13.

MINISTRY OF HEALTH 1993d. Memo from Evan Voyce, Crown Health Enterprises Establishment Unit to various officials.

MINISTRY OF HEALTH 1993e. Notes of Meeting Re: Post Election Briefing, CHEMU Various officials. HC 27-00-19-0.

MINISTRY OF HEALTH 1993f. Post Election Briefing – Draft Paper Outline. HC 27-00-19-0.

MINISTRY OF HEALTH 1993g. Report of Focus Groups. HC 03-05-01.

MINISTRY OF HEALTH 1996.

MINISTRY OF HEALTH c1992. Rod Carr, Convenor of the Prime Ministerial Committee on the Implementation of the Social Assistance Reforms. HC 28-28-0.

MINISTRY OF HEALTH n.d.-a. 'Contracting for Personal Health Services' Transition. HC 28-36.

MINISTRY OF HEALTH n.d.-b. A Report to the Minister of Health on the Implementation of Charging. HC 28-40-0#1.

MINISTRY OF HEALTH FILES 1991. Draft Memorandum for Cabinet Prime Ministerial Committee on Reform of Social Assistance. Wellington.

MINISTRY OF HEALTH FILES 1992a. HRD Cabinet Papers – Social Assistance Reform Committee – Agenda and Minute Papers Cabinet. Wellington.

MINISTRY OF HEALTH FILES 1992b. Memo from Health Reforms Directorate: Health Reforms Stocktake from Minister of Health and Michael Wintringham, Convenor, Health Reforms Management Group. Wellington.

MINISTRY OF HEALTH FILES 1992c. Memo from Loraine Hawkins to David Smyth. Wellington.

MINISTRY OF HEALTH FILES 1992d. Memo from Paul Gini from Phil Barry. Wellington.

MINISTRY OF HEALTH FILES 1992e. Memo to David Smyth from Phil Barry. Wellington.

MINISTRY OF HEALTH FILES 1992f. Memo to David Smyth from Victor Klap. Wellington.

MINISTRY OF HEALTH FILES 1992g. Memo to Minister of Finance from Loraine Hawkins, Re: ITR. Wellington.

MINISTRY OF HEALTH FILES 1992h. Memorandum to Chairmen Cabinet Committee on Social Assistance Reforms: Principles and processes for determining the health budget during and after reforms. Wellington.

MINISTRY OF HEALTH FILES 1992i. Questions from PMs Department answered by M. Goddard, Treasury Wellington.

MINISTRY OF HEALTH FILES 1992j. Treasury Report to Minister of Finance from Loraine Hawkins, Health User Charges: Long Term Strategy. Wellington.

MINISTRY OF HEALTH FILES 1993. Letter from DG MOH to Various Ministers. HC 27-00-0.

NATIONAL ADVISORY COMMITTEE ON HEALTH AND DISABILITIES 1996. Newsletter. *National Health Committee News and Issues.* National Advisory Committee on Health and Disabilities.

NATIONAL ARCHIVES 1987. Health Sector Taskforce ABQU 632 W4452 1087 63153.

NATIONAL ARCHIVES 1991a. Minutes and Project Planning for the Review of Benefits and Interim Targeting. ABQU 632 W4452 70285.

NATIONAL ARCHIVES 1991b. Reform of Social Assistance: Indicative Timeline. ABQU 632 W4452 2079 27875.

NATIONAL ARCHIVES 1991c. Rod Carr Fax to Loraine Hawkins. ABQU 632 W4452 2079 72785.

NATIONAL ARCHIVES c1991. Health Services Taskforce – General – Constitution Appendix One: Draft Letter of Referral from Prime Minister to the Minister of Health. ABQU 632 W4452 387 72784.

NATIONAL INTERIM PROVIDER BOARD 1992. Report to the Government and the New Zealand Public. Wellington, National Interim Provider Board.

NEW ZEALAND DEPARTMENT OF HEALTH 1992. *Policy Guidelines to Regional Health Authorities*. Wellington, Ministry of Health.

ORR, R. 1997. *Rural Hospitals: the Politics of Institutional Change in the Health Sector.* Master of Arts, University of Canterbury.

KLEIN, R. 1996. 'Self-inventing Institutions: Institutional Design and the U.K. Welfare State'. *In:* GOODIN, R.E. (ed.) *The Theory of Institutional Design.* New York, Cambridge University Press.

SKOCPOL, T. 1996. *Boomerang: Clinton's Health Security Effort and the Turn Against Government in U.S. Politic.* New York, W.W. Norton & Co.

STEERING GROUP ON THE IMPLEMENTATION OF THE COALITION AGREEMENT 1997. Steering Group Report. Wellington, Steering Group.

UMR INSIGHT 1993–1996a. Survey Question: In your view have the government's health reforms overall been a success or a failure? [N=750, Margin of Error: +/- 3.5%]. Wellington, UMR Insight.

UMR INSIGHT 1993–1996b. Surveys. Wellington, UMR Research Ltd.

VOWLES, J. & AIMER, P. 1993. *Voters' Vengeance : The 1990 Election in New Zealand and the Fate of the Fourth Labour Government.* Auckland, Auckland University Press.

WEAVER, R. K. 1986. The Politics of Blame Avoidance. *Journal of Public Policy,* 6.

CHAPTER SEVEN. The rise and demise of the Health Funding Authority

COALITION AGREEMENT 1996. *Coalition Agreement Between New Zealand First and the New Zealand National Party, 11 December.* Wellington, Coalition Government.

CREECH, W. 1999. *The Government's Medium-term Strategy for Health and Disability Support Services 1999.* Wellington, Ministry of Health.

DONELAN, K., BLENDON, R., SCHOEN, C., DAVIS, K. & BINNS, K. 1999. The Cost of Health System Change: Public Discontent in Five Nations. *Health Affairs,* 18, 206–216.

EVENING POST 2000. Labour to Abolish Market-led Health Model, 17.

GAULD, R. 2003. The Impact on Officials of Public Sector Restructuring: The Case of the New Zealand Health Funding Authority. *International Journal of Public Sector Management,* 16, 303–319.

GAULD, R. 2009. *Revolving Doors: New Zealand's Health Reforms – The Continuing Saga.* Wellington, Institute of Policy Studies and Health Services Research Centre.

GAULD, R. & DERRETT, S. 2000. Solving the Surgical Waiting List Problem? New Zealand's 'Booking System'. *International Journal of Health Planning and Management,* 15, 259–272.

GOLDFINCH, S. 1998. Remaking New Zealand's Economic Policy: Institutional Elites as Radical Innovators 1984–1993. *Governance,* 11, 177–207.

HAM, C. 1997. Reforming the New Zealand Health Reforms. *British Medical Journal,* 314, 1844–1845.

HAWKINS, L. & VAITHIANATHAN, R. 1997. *Accountability Mechanisms for the National Funding Agency and its Relationship with the Ministry of Health, Report commissioned by Graham Scott.* Unpublished document.

HEALTH FUNDING AUTHORITY 1998a. *The Next Five Years in General Practice.* Wellington, Health Funding Authority.

HEALTH FUNDING AUTHORITY 1998b. *Prioritisation Methodology and Process.* Wellington, Health Funding Authority.

HEALTH FUNDING AUTHORITY 1998c. *Transformation 98: Detailed Design Proposal.* Wellington, Health Funding Authority.

HEALTH FUNDING AUTHORITY 1999. *Briefing Papers for the Incoming Minister of Health.* Wellington, Health Funding Authority.

HEALTH FUNDING AUTHORITY 2000. *Improving Our Health: The Challenge for New Zealand.* Wellington, Health Funding Authority.

MĀORI HEALTH COMMISSION 1999. *Tihei Mauri Ora!* Wellington, The Māori Health Commission.

MARTIN, J. 1997. Health Structures and the Coalition. *Health Manager,* 4, 3–5.

MCKENZIE WEBSTER 1997a. *Analysis of CHE Deficits Issues: Report for the Transitional Health Authority.* Wellington, McKenzie Webster Consultants.

MCKENZIE WEBSTER 1997b. *Issues with Funding, Models, Management and Accountability Matters in Relation to RHAs, CHEs, and Central Agencies. Report prepared for Graham Scott.* Wellington, McKenzie Webster Consultants.

MINISTRY OF HEALTH 1996a. *Healthy New Zealanders: Briefing Papers for the Minister of Health.* Wellington, Ministry of Health.

MINISTRY OF HEALTH 1996b. *Sustainable Funding Package for the Health and Disability Sector.* Wellington, Ministry of Health.

MINISTRY OF HEALTH 1997. *The Evergreen (Funding) Document 1 August 1997.* Wellington, Ministry of Health.

MINISTRY OF HEALTH 1998. *Strategic Business Plan, 1997–2002.* Wellington, Ministry of Health.

MINISTRY OF HEALTH 1999. *The Health and Disability Sector: General Briefing for Hon Wyatt Creech Minister of Health.* Wellington, Ministry of Health.

MINISTRY OF HEALTH 2000. *Health Funding Authority Performance Report Quarter Three 1999–2000.* Wellington, Ministry of Health.

NATIONAL HEALTH COMMITTEE 1997. *When to Consult Communities.* Wellington, National Health Committee.

SCOTT, G., BUSHNELL, P. & SALLEE, N. 1990. Reform of the Core Public Sector: New Zealand Experience. *Governance,* 3, 138–167.

SHIPLEY, J. 1995. Advancing Health in New Zealand. Wellington: Minister of Health.

STEERING GROUP 1997. *Implementing the Coalition Agreement on Health. The report of the Steering Group to oversee health and disability changes to the Minister of Health and Associate Minister of Health.* Wellington, Steering Group.

STENT, R. 1998. *Canterbury Health Limited: A Report by the Health and Disability Commissioner April.* Wellington, Health and Disability Commissioner.

TREASURY 1996. *Briefing to the Incoming Government.* Wellington, Government Printer.

2000. New Zealand Public Health and Disability Act 2000. New Zealand: http://www.legislation.govt.nz

BARNETT, P. & CLAYDEN, C. 2007. *Governance in District Health Boards.* Wellington, Health Services Research Centre, Victoria University of Wellington.

BARNETT, P., TENBENSEL, T., CUMMING, J., CLAYDEN, C., ASHTON, T., PLEDGER, M. & BURNETTE, M. 2009. Implementing New Modes of Governance in the New Zealand Health System: An Empirical Study. *Health Policy,* 93, 118–127.

BEN TOVIM, D., BASSHAM, J., BENNETT, D., DOUGHERTY, M., MARTIN, M., O'NEILL, S., SINCOCK, J. & SZWARCBORD, M. 2008. Redesigning Care at the Flinders Medical Centre: Clinical Process Redesign Using 'Lean Thinking'. *Medical Journal of Australia,* 188, s27–s31.

BIRCHFIELD, R. & MUELLER, J. 2010. Ailing DHB Directors: Tony Ryall's Health Sector Tonic. *New Zealand Management,* March, 30–34.

BLAKELY, T., TOBIAS, M., ATKINSON, J., YEH, L.C. & HUANG, K. 2007. *Tracking Disparity: Trends in Ethnic and Socioeconomic Inequalities in Mortality, 1981–2004.* Wellington, Ministry of Health.

CHAUDRY, B., WANG, J., WU, S., MAGLIONE, M., MOJICA, W., ROTH, E., MORTON, S. & SHEKELLE, P. 2006. Systematic Review: Impact of Health Information Technology on Quality, Efficiency, and Costs of Medical Care. *Annals of Internal Medicine,* 144, 742–752.

CRUMP, B. & ADIL, M. 2009. Can Quality and Productivity Improve in a Financially Poorer NHS? *British Medical Journal,* 339, 1175–1177.

DAVIS, P., LAY-YEE, R., BRIANT, R., ALI, W., SCOTT, A. & SCHUG, S. 2002. Adverse Events in New Zealand Public Hospitals: Occurrence and Impact. *New Zealand Medical Journal,* 115, 1167.

DESAI, J. 2012. Whither Hospital Productivity in New Zealand? Estimates of Productivity and Efficiency of Public Hospitals in New Zealand (2007-09). Presentation to Health Services Research Centre 17 May. Wellington, Health Services Research Centre, Victoria University of Wellington.

EXWORTHY, M., BERNEY, L. & POWELL, M. 2002. How Great Expectations in Westminster may be Dashed Locally: The Local Implementation of National Policy on Health Inequalities. *Policy and Politics,* 30, 79–96.

FARRELL, D.M. 2001. *Electoral Systems: A Comparative Introduction.* Basingstoke, Palgrave.

GAULD, R. 2008. The Unintended Consequences of New Zealand's Primary Care Reforms. *Journal of Health Politics, Policy and Law,* 33, 93–117.

HEALTH AND DISABILITY COMMISSIONER 2007. *Capital and Coast District Health Board. A Report by the Health and Disability Commissioner (Case 05HDC11908).* Auckland, Health and Disability Commissioner.

HEALTH COMMITTEE 2006. *2006/07 Estimates Vote Health. Report of the Health Committee.* Wellington, House of Representatives.

HEFFORD, M. & DE BOER, M. 2003. Service Planning and Prioritisation in a

District Health Board. *In:* GAULD, R. (ed.) *Continuity Amid Chaos: Health Care Management and Delivery in New Zealand.* Dunedin: University of Otago Press.

KING, A. 2000. *The New Zealand Health Strategy.* Wellington, Minister of Health.

KING, A. 2001. *The Primary Health Care Strategy.* Wellington, Ministry of Health.

MALCOLM, L., WRIGHT, L. & BARNETT, P. 1999. *The Development of Primary Care Organisations in New Zealand: A Review Undertaken for Treasury and the Ministry of Health.* Wellington, Ministry of Health.

MAYS, N., CUMMING, J. & TENBENSEL, T. 2007. *Health Reforms 2001 Research: Overview Report.* Wellington, Health Services Research Centre.

MINISTERIAL REVIEW GROUP 2009. *Meeting the Challenge: Enhancing Sustainability and the Patient and Consumer Experience within the Current Legislative Framework for Health and Disability Services in New Zealand.* Wellington, Minister of Health.

MINISTRY OF HEALTH 2000. *District Health Board Establishment: Final Planning Guidelines.* Wellington, Ministry of Health.

MINISTRY OF HEALTH 2008a. *2007/08 Annual Report on Indicators of DHB Performance (IDP).* Wellington, Ministry of Health.

MINISTRY OF HEALTH 2008b. *Briefing for the Incoming Minister of Health.* Wellington, Ministry of Health.

MINISTRY OF HEALTH 2008c. *Health Targets. Moving Towards Healthier Futures, 2007/08 – The Results.* Wellington, Ministry of Health.

OECD 2009. *Health at a Glance 2009.* Paris, Organisation for Economic Cooperation and Development.

QUALITY IMPROVEMENT COMMITTEE 2009. *Sentinel and Serious Events in New Zealand Hospitals 2007–2008.* Wellington, The Quality Improvement Committee.

STARFIELD, B., SHI, L. & MACINKO, J. 2005. Contribution of primary care to health systems and health. *The Milbank Quarterly,* 83, 457–502.

TREASURY 2005. *Value for Money in Health – The DHB Sector.* Wellington, The Treasury.

WHITEHEAD, M., HANRATTY, B. & POPAY, J. 2010. NHS Reform: Untried Remedies for Misdiagnosed Problems? *The Lancet,* 376, 1373–1375.

CHAPTER NINE. Conclusion: realism and representation

ARNOLD, R.D. 1990. *The Logic of Congressional Action.* New Haven, Yale University Press.

ARNSTEIN, S. 1969. A Ladder of Participation. *Journal of the American Institute of Planners,* 35, 4, 216–223.

BARNARD, C.I. 1938. *The Functions of the Executive.* Cambridge, Mass., Harvard University Press.

BUSH, G.W.A. 1980. *Local Government and Politics in New Zealand.* Sydney and Boston, George Allen & Unwin.

DEPARTMENT OF HEALTH 1975. *A Health Service for New Zealand.* Wellington, Government Printer.

DORGAN, S., LAYTON, D., BLOOM, N., HOMKES, R., SADUN, R. & VAN REENEN, J. 2010. *Management in Healthcare: Why Good Practice Really Matters.* London, McKinsey and Co.

EVENING POST 2000. Labour to Abolish Market-led Health Model, 2 August, 17.

FEREJOHN, J.A. 1990. Information and the Electoral Process. *In:* FEREJOHN, J. A. & KUKLINSKI, J. H. (eds.) *Information and Democratic Processes.* Urbana, Illinois, University of Illinois.

FLORIN, D. & DIXON, J. 2004. Public Involvement in Health Care. *British Medical Journal,* 328, 159–161.

FUDGE, N., WOLFE, C.D.A. & MCKEVITT, C. 2008. Assessing the Promise of User Involvement in Health Service Development: Ethnographic Study. *British Medical Journal,* 336, 313–317.

GOODALL, A.H. 2011. Physician-leaders and Hospital Performance: Is there an Association? *Social Science & Medicine,* 73, 535–539.

HAM, C. & ROBERT, G. (eds.) 2003. *Reasonable Rationing: International Experience of Priority Setting in Health Care.* Buckingham: Open University Press.

HIRSCHMAN, A.O. 1970. *Exit, Voice, and Loyalty: Responses to Decline in Firms, Organizations, and States.* Cambridge, Mass., Harvard University Press.

JACOBS, L.R. 1993. *The Health of Nations.* Ithaca, Cornell University Press.

JAMES, B.C. & SAVITZ, L.A. 2011. How Intermountain Trimmed Health Care Costs through Robust Quality Improvement Efforts. *Health Affairs,* 30, 1185–1191.

JHA, A. & EPSTEIN, A. 2010. Hospital Governance and the Quality of Care. *Health Affairs,* 29, 182–7.

MORRELL, W.P. 1964 [1932]. *The Provincial System in New Zealand 1852–76.* Christchurch, Whitcombe and Tombs.

MULGAN, R. G. 1984. *Democracy and Power in New Zealand: A Study of New Zealand Politics.* Auckland, Oxford University Press.

NATIONAL ARCHIVES 1987. What do Hospitals Provide Other than Just Care? What are Consumers' Expectations? Memo to the Taskforce on Hospital and Related Services by M.E. Holman. Wellington: National Archives ABQU W4452 632 64416.

NATIONAL ARCHIVES 1988. Letters to Consultants – Fraser, Gibbs, Scott, From Ministers of Health and Finance. ABQU W4452 632 1090 64410.

NATIONAL HEALTH BOARD & SOUTHERN DISTRICT HEALTH BOARD 2011. Joint Assessment of Systems, Dunedin Hospital. Wellington: National Health Board.

OLIVER, W.H. 1977. The Origins and Growth of the Welfare State. *In:* TRLIN, A.D. (ed.) *Social Welfare and New Zealand Society.* Wellington: Methuen Publications.

PEMBER-REEVES, W. [1898] 1950. *The Long White Cloud: Ao Tea Roa.* London, George Allen & Unwin.

PITKIN, H.F. 1972. *The Concept of Representation.* Berkeley, CA: University of California Press.

SELZNICK, P. 1957. *Leadership in Administration: A Sociological Interpretation.* New York, Harper & Row.

STEERING GROUP ON THE IMPLEMENTATION OF THE COALITION AGREEMENT 1997. Steering Group Report. Wellington: Steering Group.

SUTCH, W.B. 1956. Local Government in New Zealand: A History of Defeat. *In:* POLASCHEK, R. J. (ed.) *Local Government in New Zealand*. Wellington: New Zealand Institute of Public Administration.

Index

access to health care 22, 32, 46, 51, 76, 86, 90, 117, 118, 125, 134, 136, 142, 152, 153–4, 157, 168, 169, 173, 175

accountability: Area Health Boards 99, 104; Crown Health Enterprises 112, 125–6; District Health Boards 12, 140, 141, 142, 149; dual accountability to central government and local communities 12, 99, 104, 141, 149, 160, 170, 171; and efficiency 59, 125–6, 128–9; general practitioners 87; hospital boards 18, 100; hospitals 59, 61, 87, 90; and market system 84; Minister of Health's advocacy for 98; for public health 99; Regional Health Authorities 112, 125–6; and representation 10, 169–70, 171; types of 26

advisory boards in health care 77

Alliance Party 116, 125, 137–8

Americanisation of New Zealand health care system 108, 121

Area Health Boards (AHBs) 13, 14, 27, 78–9, 86, 91, 93, 94, 96, 116, 122; accountability 99, 104; conflict between local accountability and central funding 99, 104; contracting with providers 86, 93; elected members 118; elected/appointed member mix 78, 81, 93–4, 101, 102; elimination of elected membership 14, 28, 101, 102, 104–5, 107, 119, 120, 121, 122, 165, 174; functions and responsibilities 79–80, 85; funding 98, 99; and health outcomes 99; performance contracts 99; and primary health care 93, 98; and public health 99; as a safety net 94, 97

Area Health Boards Act 1983 27, 79, 100

Area Health Boards Amendment Act 1989 81, 82, 99

Arnstein's 'ladder of participation' 25, 171

Arthur Andersen and Company 92

Associated Chambers of Commerce 49

Auckland 15, 16, 65, 70, 173

Australia 22, 32, 34, 84, 162; hospital governance and organisation 35, 41–2

Barnard, W.E. 50

Barrowclough, H.E. 57 see also Consultative Committee on Health Reform 1953 (Barrowclough Commission)

Bassett, Michael 83, 86, 89

Begg, Campbell 49

benefit selection 93
benefits, *see* health benefits; hospital
   benefits; pharmaceutical benefits;
   welfare state
Beveridge-style systems 32–3
Bismarckian systems 32
Board of Health 84
Bristol Royal Infirmary Inquiry 23
Britain 31, 32, 34, 64, 110, 121,
   162–4, 174; hospital governance and
   organisation 35, 36–7, 42; *see also*
   England; National Health Service
   (NHS); Scotland
British Medical Association (New
   Zealand Branch) (BMA) 50, 51, 53,
   58, 72 *see also* Medical Association of
   New Zealand (MANZ)
Bryce, Jessie 47
budget-holding 125

Cabinet Social Equity Committee 96
Canada 10, 25, 34; hospital governance
   and organisation 35, 38–9
Capital Coast District Health Board
   145, 152
Capital Development Committee 157
capitation model 53, 70, 85, 125
Caygill, David 86, 87, 92, 93, 96, 98, 99;
   'Health: A Prescription for Change'
   98
centralisation/decentralisation of health
   services 33–5, 172–5; decision-
   making 34–5, 65, 159, 160; dual
   accountability to central government
   and local communities 99, 104, 141,
   149, 160; in federal health systems
   34, 35, 38, 40, 41–2; Gibbs Taskforce
   93, 94, 97; hospital governance
   35–43; in national health systems 34,
   35; *see also* geographic organisation
   of health system; regionalisation;
   regionalisation, New Zealand
CHEs, *see* Crown Health Enterprises
   (CHEs)
Chief Nurses of New Zealand 86
child health services 74, 114, 119, 127;
   free doctor visits and medicines,
   children under 6 117, 127

Christchurch ward, Canterbury District
   Health Board 145
citizen participation, *see* public
   participation
Clark, Helen 99
clinical governance 22–4, 156, 157, 168,
   170, 174; skills and expertise 151
'Coalition Agreement on Health'
   117–18, 125–9, 131; Steering Group
   127–8, 130
collaboration between government
   agencies 128, 134, 137, 168
collectivism 89
commercialisation of providers 93, 94,
   95, 96, 101, 102, 105, 107–8
communications strategies 109–10, 115,
   121, 127–8; District Health Board
   elections 143–4; information about
   health care system 138, 140; service
   costing and funding information 133
communities: and Area Health Boards
   79, 99; boards' dual accountability
   to central government and local
   communities 12, 99, 104, 141, 149,
   160, 170, 171; communication
   about health reforms 109–10, 115,
   119, 121, 127–8, 133; community
   action centres 76; control of, and
   ties to, local hospitals 162, 163–6,
   167; European settlement 162–3;
   influence on spatial distribution of
   services or governance 33, 34–5, 42–3,
   61, 80; needs, and funding of health
   services 32–3, 79, 135, 142–3, 151,
   170, 171; preferences 94, 120, 163,
   165, 171, 172; responsiveness to 12,
   64, 84, 102, 104, 107, 119, 175; *see
   also* centralisation/decentralisation of
   health services; consumers; elected
   health boards; public opinion; public
   participation; representation
communities of interest 33, 59, 76
community partnership 10
competition in health services provision
   and financing 14, 22, 36, 92, 93, 95,
   99, 101, 102, 103, 105; 'Coalition
   Agreement on Health' 125, 128–9;
   Crown Health Enterprises 111;

failure to deliver efficiency savings 13, 117, 120, 125–6; within framework of publicly managed and financed services 121; gains from 125, 133; Health Benefits Review 81, 83, 85, 87; Health Funding Authority 28, 131, 132; insurance markets 93, 113, 119; managed 106; and purchaser-provider split 111–12; Regional Health Authorities 118, 119; shift away from 120, 124, 125, 128, 159; survival of policy 118; tendering 126; *see also* market-oriented health services

consultation 25, 26, 52, 57–8, 71, 73, 76, 77, 94, 114, 119, 134, 137–8, 171; District Health Boards 137–8, 140, 142–3, 150; *see also* public participation

Consultative Committee on Health Reform 1953 (Barrowclough Commission) 14, 26, 57–60, 61, 70

consumer-funding model 91

consumers: choice 56, 76, 83, 85, 88, 92, 93, 102; groups 79, 80; and health reform 64, 74, 83, 90, 91, 93, 102, 104 *see also* communities; public opinion; public participation

contestability 115

contracting/purchasing 14, 27, 36, 117, 125, 130–1; Area Health Boards 93; centralised 28; collaborative 128, 132, 135; District Health Boards 14, 142; 'evergreen' contracts 133; Health Benefits Review 81, 86; and health outcomes 126, 132–3; Ministry of Health 142, 153; national frameworks 135; Regional Health Authorities 103, 104, 111, 116–17, 118, 126, 132; Steering Group, Coalition Agreement on Health 128; *see also* funding and expenditure; Health Funding Authority (HFA); purchaser-provider split

co-payments 87, 93, 101, 105–6, 110, 113–14, 117, 118, 120, 155

core health services 114–15, 118, 119, 128

Core Services Committee 114–15, 138 *see also* National Health Committee

corporate governance model 13, 21, 22, 124, 172

Counties Manukau District Health Board 145

Creech, Wyatt 134

Cropper, James Richard 67

Crown Company Monitoring Advisory Unit (CCMAU) 125

Crown Health Enterprises (CHEs) 111, 112–13, 117–18, 119–20, 125–6, 130; funding 112, 127, 130; intervention by ministers 112; profit objectives 112, 117, 118, 123; public resistance to 111, 112; *see also* Hospital and Health Services (HHSs); hospitals

Crown Health Enterprises Minister 112–13

Culyer, Anthony 92–3

Dannevirke Hospital Board 58, 66

decentralisation of health services, *see* centralisation/decentralisation of health services

decision-making: decentralisation 34–5, 65, 159, 160; democratic 24; elected health boards 10; public participation 10, 21–2, 24–6, 28, 35, 76, 78, 94, 120, 124, 128, 134, 137, 140, 142, 165, 171

democracy: decision-making 24; democratic governance 9, 21–2, 139, 143–4, 150, 159, 164, 165, 167, 168, 174–5; hospital board embodiment of community values 19

Department of Health 29; and Area Health Boards 78–9; and blueprint for reform, 1991 102–3; district offices replaced by health boards 77, 79; and Gibbs Taskforce 83, 88, 92; and health insurance 50; and hospital boards 56, 58–9, 64–5, 90, 167; and hospital system 64–5, 163; and Hospitals Advisory Council 60; and Labour Caucus Committee on Health 69, 70; and local representation 27, 70; mental health institution

transition to Area Health Boards 79, 82, 98, 99, 100; *see also* health boards
Hospital Boards' Association 18, 29, 47–8, 49, 50, 51, 52, 57, 73, 79, 98
hospital districts 15, 17; amalgamation 48–50, 56, 57, 64, 141; *see also* health districts
hospitals: access to public hospitals 19, 46, 47; accountability 59, 61, 87, 90; beds *per capita*, 1969 65, 66; closures 20, 27, 37, 43, 57, 60, 65, 68, 90, 109, 164, 165; commercialisation 93, 94, 95, 96, 101, 102, 105, 107–8, 112; control and management 15–16, 18–19, 22, 35–43, 52, 53, 54, 56–60, 61, 64, 65, 70, 95, 138, 160, 162, 163, 164, 167–8; co-payment for services 101, 105–6, 117, 118; cross-national governance and organisation 35–43; Department of Health survey, 1969 65; and District Health Boards 142; efficiency 27, 152–3; emergency department visit charges 106, 113, 150; emergency department waiting times 156; establishment during gold rush period 15; fees 46, 47–8, 50; financial pressures 47, 127, 170; free care 18, 26, 47, 54, 90, 152; funding and expenditure 12, 26, 45–6, 48–9, 51, 54–5, 56, 57, 59–60, 77, 152–3, 161, 168; medical practice variation 24; patient charges 101, 105–6, 113, 117, 118, 150; patient safety 22–4, 127, 132, 138, 158, 173; privatisation 94–5, 96, 98, 100, 107, 167; provision of care 16, 47; public and parliamentary oversight 138; public opinion 86, 108; public share issues 94; regionalisation of small, local hospitals 13, 27, 34, 48–50, 56–60, 61, 68; social reputation 46; throughput increases 125; waiting lists 69, 86, 104, 117, 125, 127, 133, 136, 153–4; *see also* Crown Health Enterprises (CHEs); Hospital and Health Services (HHSs)
Hospitals Act 1957 15, 17, 19, 26–7, 59
Hospitals Advisory Council 27, 60

Hospitals Amendment Act 1951 55
Hutchinson, Charles Pierrepont 67
Hutt Valley District Health Board 142–3

Illich, Ivan 64
incrementalism 11–12, 76, 80, 100
Independent Practitioner Associations 135, 136, 158
inequity, *see* equity
infectious diseases 16
information dissemination, *see* communications strategies
information technology (IT): decisions 34–5; national consistency and standards 157; skills and expertise 151
institutional knowledge 127, 128, 130, 131, 132
institutions 11
insurance, private 40, 73, 80, 86, 93, 96, 101, 102, 105, 109, 116, 118, 119, 120
insurance programmes 32, 33, 37, 39, 40, 42, 65, 91, 92, 93, 95, 96, 118, 168; *see also* national health insurance; social insurance
Integrated Family Health Centre 158
interest groups 12, 68, 69, 71, 72–5, 77, 79, 80, 84, 96, 100, 102

Japan 32

King, Annette 137, 168
Kirton, Neil 129–30

Labour Caucus Committee on Health 14, 69, 70
Labour Governments: First, 1935–49 19, 26, 45–6, 51–4, 60, 69–70, 71; Second, 1957–60; Third, 1972–75 14, 27, 63, 68–75, 80; ; Fourth, 1984–90 13, 27–8, 81–100, 121, 167
Labour-led Governments 28, 124–5, 137, 138, 139, 140–4, 148–9, 152, 154, 159, 167, 168
Labour Party 89, 95, 97–8, 100, 116, 159, 167
Lange, David 83, 97, 98, 100, 167